Developing and Organizing an Institutional
Biospecimen Repository

Donna E. Hansel, MD, PhD
Scott D. Jewell, PhD
Editors

cap PRESS
Northfield, Illinois

Library of Congress Control Number: 2014937501
ISBN: 9780983706854

Printed in the USA

College of American Pathologists
325 Waukegan Road
Northfield, Illinois 60093
800-323-4040
cap.org

Contents

Preface

Donna E. Hansel
Scott D. Jewell

Scientific investigation utilizing human tissue requires specimens to be (1) representative of the disease process, (2) consistently of good to excellent quality, (3) of adequate size and volume for research, and (4) annotated with sufficient clinical data and demographics to ensure high value and usability in most research.

Biospecimen quality and usability has varied significantly within and across institutions, which has prompted improvement in standard operating procedures for biospecimen collection and biobanking. Some of the hallmark standards include greater attention and action to acquire informed consent from patients for the donation and use of biospecimens; timely collection and processing procedures for biospecimens; efficient, accurate, and well-documented cost-lowering processes in biobanking management; and consistent, ethical, and regulatory management for the distribution and use of tissues in research. The establishment of the International Society of Biological and Environmental Repositories (ISBER) in 1999 and the Biorepositories and Biospecimen Research Branch (BBRB; formerly the Office of Biorepositories and Biospecimen Research [OBBR]) established by the National Cancer Institute in 2005, as well as several European groups (Biobanking and Biomolecular Resources Research Infrastructure [BBMRI] and European, Middle Eastern and African Society for Biopreservation and Biobanking [ESBB]), have lead to the development of best practices and guidelines to improve procedures in biobanking, which are used throughout the world. The lessons learned to date can be applied broadly to all biospecimen and tissue-based studies. However, the direction towards more stringent requirements are still needed for the collection, processing, banking, and distribution of human biospecimens for research because the findings in research need to relate more accurately to the precision of clinical medicine. In 2012, the College of American Pathologists (CAP) launched a Biorepository Accreditation Program that will assist biorepositories that want to meet strict process and procedure criteria through a peer review process.

The purpose of this publication is to provide information on establishing and maintaining a biospecimen repository and to discuss issues critical to proper specimen usage. Topics such as patient-informed consent, quality control, ethics, and information systems are discussed in detail. While biospecimens can encompass all human biological material used for research or medical practice, the main focus of discussion in this book will be directed to tissues, especially those that may be procured through routine clinical procedures or the clinical or anatomic pathology services. Although best practices for biorepositories and all factors associated with biorepositories are still in development at the national and international level, we have provided current information to the reader from the lessons we have learned.

The use of human tissue specimens for research has gained increasing attention, in part because of the intense competition within and outside of academic institutions, genetic identifiability, ethical issues regarding ownership, and the development of personalized health care. These issues have led to a surge in defining the conditions under which biospecimen repositories are developed and operate, including patient-informed consent, biospecimen processing and quality control, completeness of annotated medical information, informatics, access, and sustainability. Conceptually, high-quality biospecimens (with biological and medical annotation) provide the best data for proper interpretation of research results. Historically, tissue biobanking has been undertaken by a small number of researchers and pathologists interested in using specimens for defined individual research purposes. However, increasing awareness of the importance of proper biospecimen management has led to rapid developments, with many institutions and agencies defining priorities and guidelines for biospecimen banking. In-depth analysis of the management of these specimens has led to expansion of the biobanking enterprise into biospecimen science, common consent procedures, ethical standards, compatible applications and databases, ease of sharing biospecimens with patient medical information annotation, and oversight committees to manage conflict-of-interest issues, fair tissue allocation, and extramural contracts. Development of an institutional core facility surrounding the biospecimen repository has necessitated the expansion of the infrastructure for laboratory services such as histology, immunohistochemistry, and molecular derivative processing, among others, and the development of timely cost recovery mechanisms to support these efforts. Ultimately, the growth of these institutional biorepositories, designed to promote high-quality, reproducible research using readily available biospecimens, has led to a vast array of institutional considerations that span the research, legal, and financial realms.

Why is the information needed? How will it be used? How does it relate to the CAP?

Most recently, biospecimen repositories have and will continue to receive greater attention in the field of translational medical research, which will require the involvement of diagnostic pathologists and laboratories for biospecimen collection and repository organization and maintenance. Biospecimen repositories will set the stage for large collections of patient specimens that will accelerate findings for personalized health care. This book is designed to be a key reference for those responsible for the establishment and maintenance of these biorepositories and associated core laboratories, which should be managed by pathology departments. The recruitment of key authors from diverse professional backgrounds and institutions who are knowledgeable in the field of biobanking enhances the utility of this book and provides readers with a comprehensive framework with which to implement biobanking strategies. Because the CAP represents a well-established and highly regarded body within the pathology community, this collaborative publication will allow the field of pathology to help guide the future direction of biobanking initiatives, with a potential for advancements to be made in clinical diagnoses and treatments.

Acronyms List

AACC: American Association for Clinical Chemistry

AACR: American Association for Cancer Research

ARRA: American Recovery and Reinvestment Act

ASCO: American Society of Clinical Oncology

ASCP: American Society for Clinical Pathology

BBMRI: Biobanking and Biomolecular Resources Research Infrastructure

BBRB: Biorepositories and Biospecimen Research Branch

BDUA: Biorepository Distribution and Use Agreement

BRD: Biospecimen Research Database

BRN: Biospecimen Research Network

CAP: College of American Pathologists

CBM: Common Biorepository Model

CDMS: clinical data management system

CHTN: Cooperative Human Tissue Network

CITI: Collaborative Institutional Training Initiative

CLIA: Clinical Laboratory Improvement Amendments

DAC: Data Access Committee

ERC: Ethics Review Committee

ESBB: European, Middle Eastern and African Society for Biopreservation and Biobanking

EVS: Enterprise Vocabulary Services

FDA: US Food and Drug Administration

FFPE: formalin-fixed paraffin-embedded

FMA: Foundational Model of Anatomy Ontology

H&E: hematoxylin and eosin

HHS: US Department of Health and Human Services

HIPAA: Health Insurance Portability and Accountability Act of 1996

HUGO: Human Genome Organisation

HVAC: heating, ventilation, and air conditioning

IATA: International Air Transport Association

ICAO: International Civil Aviation Organization

ICD-O: International Classification of Diseases for Oncology

IRB: Institutional Review Board

ISBER: International Society for Biological and Environmental Repositories

miRNA: microRNA

MTA: Material Transfer Agreement

MUA: Material Use Agreement

NBN: National Biospecimen Network

NCI: National Cancer Institute

NIH: National Institutes of Health

OBBR: Office of Biorepositories and Biospecimen Research

OCT: optimal cutting temperature compound

OHRP: Office for Human Research Protections

OSHA: Occupational Safety and Health Administration

P3G: Public Population Project in Genomics

PHI: protected health information

QA: quality assurance

QC: quality control

RIN: RNA integrity number

SAT: Self-Assessment Tool

SOPs: standard operating procedures

SPORE: Specialized Programs of Research Excellence

SRL: Specimen Resource Locator

TMA: tissue microarray

UMLS: Unified Medical Language System

USCAP: United States & Canadian Academy of Pathology

UUID: Universally Unique Identifier

Contributors

Donna E. Hansel, MD, PhD
Division of Anatomic Pathology
UC San Diego
La Jolla, California

Scott D. Jewell, PhD
Program for Technologies & Cores
Van Andel Research Institute
Grand Rapids, Michigan

Dave W. Chesla, PA-ASCP
Universal Biorepository
Spectrum Health
Grand Rapids, Michigan

Sarah M. Dry, MD
Department of Pathology and Laboratory Medicine
UCLA Health
Los Angeles, California

Angen Liu, MD
Cleveland Clinic Foundation
Cleveland, Ohio

Nicole C. Lockhart, PhD
Division of Genomics and Society
National Human Genome Research Institute
National Institutes of Health
Bethesda, Maryland

M. Scott Lucia, MD
Department of Pathology
University of Colorado
Anschutz Medical Campus
Aurora, Colorado

Clara E. Magyar, PhD
Department of Pathology and Laboratory Medicine
UCLA Health
Los Angeles, California

Laura Monovich
Biopathology Center
The Research Institute at Nationwide Children's Hospital
Columbus, Ohio

Kimberly Myers, PhD
Deloitte Consulting LLP
Arlington, Virginia

Rakesh Nagarajan, MD, PhD
Division of Laboratory and Genomic Medicine
Washington University School of Medicine
St. Louis, Missouri

Nilsa C. Ramirez, MD
Biopathology Center
The Research Institute at Nationwide Children's Hospital
Columbus, Ohio

Daniel Rohrer, BS, MBA
Program for Technologies & Cores
Van Andel Research Institute
Grand Rapids, Michigan

Nicole J. Sieffert, BA, CCRC
Biorepository Regulatory Support
The University of Texas
MD Anderson Cancer Center
Houston, Texas

Dana Valley, BA, CAPM, CLSSGB, CPIA
Program for Technologies & Cores
Van Andel Research Institute
Grand Rapids, Michigan

Adrie van Bokhoven, PhD
Department of Pathology
University of Colorado
Anschutz Medical Campus
Aurora, Colorado

Mark A. Watson, MD, PhD
Division of Laboratory and Genomic Medicine
Washington University School of Medicine
St. Louis, Missouri

Chapter 1

Defining the Role of the Biospecimen Repository at Your Institution

Donna E. Hansel
Scott D. Jewell

Your institution may have an existing centralized biorepository of human biospecimens, scattered "satellite" biorepositories housed in research laboratories, or no system in place. Whether you are starting from scratch or modifying an existing system, it is important to take into account a number of factors to optimize both effectiveness and efficiency. This chapter will discuss how to obtain institutional "buy-in" from administrators and colleagues, and how to define the parameters and functions of your biorepository. Moreover, although a biorepository can be specific for vertebrate and invertebrate species as well as plant species, for the purpose of this book, we are only referring to repositories of biospecimens derived from humans.

Getting Started

You are probably reading this book because you are interested in developing a biospecimen repository for either institutional or personal needs, or you are modifying an existing biospecimen network at your institution. In either case, the appropriate procedures for collecting, processing, and banking biospecimens involve a lot of work and organization.

Increasingly, researchers and clinicians alike are realizing the importance of standardized specimen collection and annotation. Many have started their own collections, which may have existed for long periods of time, often initiated and justified by either (1) the interest of an individual researcher in a specific disease, (2) the interest of a group of patients in clinical trials, (3) an extended collection effort for rare disease entities, or (4) the lack of an existing centralized resource to assist in specimen collection. Often, these satellite banks may have paired body fluids with extensive patient outcome data, thereby making the biospecimens especially valuable and, as such, often engender a sense of ownership of these materials. The challenges inherent with the tissue ownership issue are not new and have been the primary basis underlying many of the well-publicized legal cases surrounding human tissue. In addition, the unwritten but implied ownership assumed by researchers is even more complicated organizationally for the institution and is an important principle for discussion when forming a centralized biorepository.

Ultimately, the success of developing a biorepository—regardless of scope or size—rests with garnering institutional support; assessing the needs, value, and existing infrastructure; and defining the scope of the project. The first half of this chapter covers these components in detail. Once these elements are in place, a plan can be developed that accounts for infrastructure, cost, personnel, logistics, and policies surrounding informed consent, collection, processing, banking, and information systems and software. These topics are covered in the second half of this chapter, with selected topics covered in greater detail in other chapters of the book.

Obtaining Institutional Support

Whether the scale of your operation will be large or small, departmental and institutional support must be in place. Although it may seem intuitive that a biospecimen repository would be beneficial to patients and researchers alike, the development of a biorepository often requires significant financial support and should include leadership and authority to mediate conflicts and develop policies that can be enforced. Developing and sustaining a biorepository that will provide value to a program or institution will take time and funding, which requires a well-managed and intentional effort to educate department chairs and college deans, as well as the institution's senior administrators. Some of the sentinel issues (not in any particular order of priority) include the following:

- Mutually agreeable purpose, goals, and plans for the development of the biorepository
- Well-written operating procedures and documents for the biorepository
- Ensuring ethical, social, and legal requirements for patients' consent for their contribution of biospecimens to prospective and future research

- Support for interaction with patients in the clinical setting
- Engagement and discussion with the Institutional Review Board (IRB) to ensure appropriate uses and documents needed for the distribution of biospecimens for research
- Collection and processing to ensure high-quality biospecimens with annotation of the patient's clinical information for basic and translational research
- Emphasis on the selection and management of software applications for the scope of the biorepository in tracking and managing biospecimens
- Physical location and infrastructure
- Providing extensive documentation on tissue collection and management when seeking approval from the Food and Drug Administration (FDA)
- Support for clinical trials
- Developing a core resource that may be available to industry on a cost-per-case basis
- Generating primary research on the quality of biospecimens to improve best practices
- Coordinating multiple research efforts across the institution into a core laboratory and biospecimen resource to reduce overall costs
- Evolving into a site that may host a cooperative group tissue collection
- Identifying opportunities to obtain grant funding that can support both infrastructure and technical development

The value of the biorepository to the institution can be measured in many ways but certainly includes some potential benefits such as a reduction in costs when processes are consolidated to support clinical trials, the ability to serve multiple-user research needs, enhancement of patent or intellectual property protection, and support of research for FDA approval of new devices or interventions. Thus, biospecimen repositories can reduce expenses while promoting quality; however, the establishment of a biorepository may require start-up and/or additional institutional funding that should be considered. Once a biorepository is established, its value to the institution would be measured by increased competitiveness in grant and contract applications, faculty recruitment, research standing and education, and, altruistically, by improvement in patient care. The scope and goals of a biobank must be planned through in-depth discussion among key scientific stakeholders and administrators. Frequently, the assessment of overall value will be questioned, with such questions as:

- How much will this cost the institution?
- How much will it cost the investigators who use biospecimens from this facility?
- Why should we spend money developing this program?

Other important points often raised in discussion include:

- How do we determine the long-term need or successful effects?
- Where will the biorepository be located?
- Who is going to manage it?

In fact, most of the costs may be recovered over time through indirect and direct grant costs and chargeback systems, but the initial start-up will require institutional investment to develop an effective biorepository.

The location of the biospecimen facility can be critical to its functionality, but a comprehensive biorepository can't be at every location for all biospecimen collection points. The majority of successful institutional biorepositories are centralized, housed in either the pathology department or the cancer center. Pathology is a logical site to establish and oversee this facility, with the close proximity to the operating rooms, tissue analysis done at the time of collection, and blood processing that is routine in the department. In addition, cancer centers periodically house the main repository if there are abundant resources available and if the primary goal of the enterprise is cancer focused. In any biorepository scenario where human tissues are collected and maintained, close involvement of the pathology department is critical to ensure that high-quality specimens are obtained, evaluated, and stored appropriately.

Chapter 2

Getting Started: Developing an Institutional Resource Within the Pathology Department

Donna E. Hansel
Angen Liu

When considering the location of a newly developed biospecimen repository, the pathology department is a logical and reasonable site in which to locate this facility. However, biospecimen repositories, also known as *biorepositories* or *biobanks,* have not usually been developed along centralized lines, and therefore the establishment of a new biorepository in light of several existing (satellite) biobanks may be somewhat challenging. The goal of this chapter is to explore the role of the pathology department in the management of biospecimens, discuss specific needs regarding specimen type, and explore the relationship between satellite versus central banks and ways in which to streamline this process.

The Pathology Department as a Central Processing and Tissue Management Hub

The pathology department is central to the collection, processing, storage, and distribution of high-quality patient specimens. These specimens range from solely frozen tissue to bodily fluids (blood, urine) to formalin-fixed paraffin-embedded (FFPE) tissue. Specific topics that require pathology assistance include the following:

- Diagnostic issues related to tissue, blood, or fluid collection
- Tissue allocation from a collected sample (gatekeeper function)
- Assessment of tissue and/or fluid quality
- Distribution of biobank tissue in conjunction with available material from patient diagnostic material

To ensure that tissue removed from patients receives the appropriate diagnostic attention, it has been recommended that all such tissue be examined by a pathologist. Specifically, before removal of a portion of the specimen for research purposes and/or biobanking, adequate gross pathology assessment is an essential part of diagnosis. Furthermore, essential portions of the specimen, such as tissue at the margin, tissue from the deepest portion of tumor invasion, and tissue from heterogeneous areas of tumor that require sampling, should be performed with accuracy to ensure an adequate final diagnosis.

After appropriate gross assessment has been performed, a portion of normal and/or tumor tissue (in the case of solid specimens) can be collected without compromising diagnosis. Although a maximum amount of tissue for biobanking purposes is desired, in limited cases 50 to 100 mg of tissue is often adequate to obtain useful DNA and RNA amounts for subsequent analysis. At the time of biospecimen collection, an adjacent section of tissue should be processed for frozen or FFPE histology analysis to assess necrosis and tissue content; in some instances, a tissue shave of the directly biobanked material can also be used for these purposes. The histologic findings are then catalogued within the informatics system used by the biorepository.

In general, frozen biobanked material is held for distribution until a final report on the diagnostic permanent material has been rendered. In the interim, it is the responsibility of the biobank facility to check biobanked material for histologic findings and relay these to the diagnostic pathologist. As an example, a frozen or FFPE section from the biobanked material should be evaluated not only to assure quality control parameters (eg, necrosis, percentage tumor) of the material, but should also be reviewed by a pathologist to ensure that all relevant information related to patient diagnosis (eg, depth of invasion, presence/absence of tumor) is relayed to the signing pathologist; rarely, the main diagnostic material may be present only in the biobanked material. It is recommended in these instances that frozen material be released for subsequent diagnostic analysis. On occasion, non-redundant tissue may be selected by a consented protocol. Such examples include an additional biopsy taken during early tumor analysis or a portion of biopsy material that is consented and submitted only for biobanking purposes. For accurate diagnosis in these instances, it is also recommended that a histologic section of biobanked material be prepared and reconciled with the final clinical diagnosis made by the pathologist. In limited specimens, recent work has suggested that performing tissue imprints of the biopsy may yield useful material for subsequent analyte analysis.[1] After material has been collected and stored, it is the purview of the biobank to assess the amount of tissue available for use; aliquot this tissue and/or fluid into appropriate amounts for whole storage or DNA, RNA, and protein analysis; and monitor how much tissue remains within the biorepository. Depending on the location, additional services, such as tissue microarray construction and research immunohistochemistry, may be incorporated into the biospecimen facility.

Adequate tissue quality is essential for reproducible and meaningful research findings derived from biobanked specimens. As such, analysis of frozen or FFPE sections of biobanked tissue (or adjacent tissue) is critical and requires pathologist interpretation. In addition, because most solid tumors are composed of a complex mixture of cells and tissue, the expertise of a pathologist to assess the percentage of necrosis, percentage of tumor cells, and type of material available within a specimen (for example, the presence of normal background tissue) is needed to determine whether a particular biobanked specimen can be used directly or whether it requires further dissection, such as the use of laser capture microdissection.[2] Depending on the core functions of an individual biorepository, DNA, RNA, and protein analysis may be performed. Pathologists are in a unique position to evaluate additional material from the patient, such as paraffin-embedded biomaterials, that may better serve a research purpose and yield more representative tissue content (in contrast to the frozen material). Finally, the pathology department is primarily responsible for storage and disposal of human specimens in compliance with state and national laws. As such, locating a central biorepository within a pathology department makes both practical and legal sense.

Storage of Biospecimens by Subtype

The three general categories of biobanked specimens (which will be considered separately, below) are as follows:

- **Solid tissue or cells,** including tissue in excess needed for diagnosis and nonredundant consented tissue obtained from directed sampling
- **Blood products,** including whole blood, plasma, serum, and buffy coat prepared from blood
- **Body fluids,** including urine, saliva, buccal swabs, and so forth

Solid tissue, derived from either normal or diseased organs, may be obtained under the auspices of redundant or nonredundant tissue protocols. In the case of redundant material, tissue in excess of that needed for diagnosis can be collected under normal gross pathology protocols and stored. In contrast, tissue collected from nonredundant specimens (eg, additional biopsies obtained from a prostate during routine sampling or a portion of a bladder transurethral resection that would otherwise be entirely submitted for diagnosis) requires additional protocols. Because this latter tissue is primarily dedicated for research purposes, a separate consent process for these directed specimens are required by most institutional review boards. Furthermore, procedures to oversee the chain of custody of these tissues should also be in place. In most instances, frozen or FFPE quality control slides of the biobanked specimen would be prepared and reviewed by a pathologist. These results would contribute to the final diagnostic pathology report and should reduce concerns about "missed diagnoses." In situations where the research protocols destroy the tissue (eg, dissociations for cell line development) or utilize a large portion of the collected tissue, the clinician and pathologist should ensure that diagnostic material is still available. Optimization of protocols to prevent warm ischemia time and thus reduce degradation of molecular derivatives is essential and may include freezing tissue within the operating or procedure room in the form of small aliquots of approximately 100 mg each. Documentation of the warm ischemia time in all cases should be attempted. Table 2-1 provides some recommendations for tissue biobanking that can optimize quality.

Another common biospecimen type consists of blood and derived blood products, including plasma, serum, and buffy coat, which may be used for analysis of germline DNA. Collection of blood samples from consented patients may be performed in association with routine clinical care and can be acquired without an additional needlestick in many cases, including procuring an extra tube during clinical blood draws or collecting from an intravenous line placed during surgery. Extraction of RNA or DNA can be performed from whole blood directly, or the blood may be processed to obtain plasma, serum, and buffy coat for cryopreservation. When plasma separation is desired, use of collection tubes containing an anticoagulant (eg, EDTA, citrate, or heparin) is recommended. In contrast, collection of serum may be optimized using tubes that are coated with no additives or with a clotting activator. For specific protein-based studies, protease inhibitors can be added to avoid extensive degradation of the proteins during sample processing. The procedures outlined in Table 2-2 are

Table 2-1. Procedures for Tissue Collection and Processing	
Preoperative Considerations	▪ Patient consent is completed before surgery. De-identified/anonymized sample may be collected if a waiver of consent has been obtained.
Operating Room	▪ Never place tissue intended for biobanking in formalin (with the exception of a quality-control section, if desired). ▪ As soon as the operative procedure allows, transport the fresh surgical specimen immediately from the surgical suite to the pathology receiving room. ▪ The specimen should be placed in a sterile container, and a patient identification sticker should be present. ▪ Ensure that the requisition form is finalized, record the excision time, and notify the pathologist and biobanking staff.
Pathology Suite	▪ Processing the tissue specimen should take place in the pathology suite. ▪ The pathologist, resident, or pathologist's assistant assesses as soon as possible if there might be tissue available for biobanking. ▪ Macroscopically describe the specimen according to routine protocol. ▪ If there appears to be excess tissue available, the pathologist, resident, or pathologist's assistant contacts the biobanking staff. ▪ Use clean utensils and work on a clean surface at all times. ▪ Separate blades should be used for sectioning tumor tissue and normal tissue to avoid cross-contamination. ▪ Dissect the specimen using clean instruments between dissection of normal and tumor tissue. ▪ Take representative parts of the specimen for routine diagnosis as priority, and decide if there is excess material available for the tissue bank. ▪ Samples selected by the pathologist are put on separate, clean surfaces, such as prelabeled dishes, for creating aliquots. ▪ Collection of normal adjacent tissue from a tumor case should be performed whenever feasible.
Biobank Personnel	▪ Upon receiving the tissues, biobank personnel assure that each specimen sample corresponds to its patient identifier. ▪ Prepare the tissue aliquots for storage on a clean surface and use clean instruments. ▪ In the ideal case, where sufficient tissue is available, a maximum of six samples (each approximately 0.5 cm^3) of every available state (if present, tumor/premalignant/normal) will be frozen. This may only be done if the diagnostic process will not be disturbed. ▪ Prepare each sample for storage on a clean surface and use clean instruments. ▪ Tissue for snap-freezing is placed in labeled cryovials and snap-frozen using liquid nitrogen. ▪ The tissue cryovials are stored at -80°C or in liquid nitrogen. Record the location and position of cryovials. ▪ Record the time of freezing. Ideally, no more than 30 minutes should elapse between time of excision and time of freezing of the tissue sample. ▪ Tissue prepared for use with optimal cutting temperature (OCT) compound and paraffin blocks should be oriented with shared cut face down for OCT/paraffin block production. – OCT block production: Place a few drops OCT into mold, orient tissue, cover tissue with OCT. Position the mold at the liquid nitrogen gas–liquid interface until the OCT becomes opaque; store at -80°C until use. – Paraffin block production: Place cassettes into fixative solution pending and proceed to the tissue processor. Routine embedding and production of a hematoxylin-and-eosin–stained slide will be used for quality assurance purpose.

suggested for blood collection and processing for biobanking.

Finally, body fluids such as urine, saliva, pancreatic juice, and various effusions may be biobanked. In many instances, collection and storage of these specimens is often investigator or protocol driven, with most fluids simply aliquoted and frozen intact. For the majority of body fluids, standardized protocols and best practices have not been developed, although methods such as enrichment for cellular content and use of cyropreservatives to prevent cell lysis may be of value, depending on the study.[3,4] In general, snap-freezing samples in liquid nitrogen may be ideal for cryopreservation of the fluid product because it has been shown to yield minimal effects on assays using some fluids, such as saliva.[5] In contrast, specimens

Table 2-2. Procedures for Blood Collection and Processing

Preoperative Considerations	▪ Patient consent is completed before blood drawn. De-identified/anonymized sample may be collected if a waiver of consent has been obtained.
Operating Room	▪ Obtain blood specimen in 1-3 anticoagulant-containing tube(s) (preferably EDTA for plasma and buffy coat fraction) and serum tube(s) coated with a clotting activator, taking note of the approximate procedure time on the requisition form. Tubes may be left at room temperature and a patient identifier sticker applied to each of them. ▪ Transport the blood sample immediately to the biobank, or contact biobank personnel to collect sample. ▪ The specimen should be placed in a sterile container to which a patient identification sticker is applied. ▪ Ensure the requisition form is finalized, record the excision time, and notify the pathologist and biobanking staff.
Biobank Personnel	▪ Upon receiving the blood sample, biobank personnel assure that each specimen sample corresponds to its patient identifier. ▪ The whole blood can be processed directly for DNA or RNA according to protocols described in other chapters. ▪ Obtain a plasma-buffy coat fraction and a serum sample for cryopreservation (instructions follow, below). ▪ **Separation of plasma from the cellular fraction** 1. Centrifuge the collection tubes that contain the blood specimen at 1500-2000*g* for 15 min at room temperature. This step will separate the blood into three visible layers: – The upper layer, which consists of plasma, is generally clear and pale yellow. – The buffy coat, or leukocyte layer, is narrow and grayish white. – The bottom layer, which consists of red blood cells (RBCs), is dark red. 2. Using an appropriate disposable transfer pipette, collect plasma, divide into aliquots, and place into labeled cryovials. 3. Collect buffy coat and wash with RBC lysis buffer to remove RBC contamination and repellet; place aliquots into labeled cryovials. 4. Collect RBCs and place aliquots into cryovials. 5. Snap-freeze all cryovials in liquid nitrogen. 6. Transfer cryovials to a storage box, and place the box immediately in the -80°C freezer or in liquid nitrogen. 7. Record location and position of the cryovials. ▪ **Separation of serum from blood samples** 1. Incubate the blood in serum tubes for 1 hour at room temperature to ensure complete coagulation. 2. After incubation, centrifuge the serum tubes at 1500*g* for 15 minutes. 3. Collect the supernatant (ie, serum), and transfer aliquots directly to the labeled cryovials. 4. Snap-freeze all cryovials in liquid nitrogen. 5. Transfer the cryovials to a storage box, and place the box immediately in the -80°C freezer or in liquid nitrogen. 6. Record location and position of the cryovials.

such as urine may require additional processing, including centrifugation or filtration, for optimal results.[6-9] Although studies on nonblood fluid storage are limited, general consensus is that storage of fluids at -80°C or in liquid nitrogen may be the best option until more detailed protocols become available.

After specimens have been collected, it is essential to incorporate appropriate clinical data and metadata into the record to allow for appropriate and insightful specimen use. Metadata collected at the time of biobanking include patient demographics, specimen size and weight, frozen section information, warm ischemia time, and pertinent information regarding gross pathology. Patient clinical data is usually captured through the use of a clinical data form or, in some systems, can be attached through an electronic linkage from the hospital research information warehouse. A copy of the consent form should be available for auditing purposes and may be held by a computer-based database system. A further discussion of information technology (IT)-based issues is covered in chapter 7, *Biorepository Informatics*.

Interaction of a Centralized Biorepository With Investigator-Based Satellite Banks

Within the same institution, two different types of biorepository may potentially exist: the central, institutionally supported biorepository; and separate, smaller, individually run satellite banks. In most cases, the concept of a centralized biorepository has been relatively recently developed. To support the cost and infrastructure of such a central facility, broad-scale institutional support has been required. In contrast, many institutions have a large number of investigator-based satellite banks. Such banks have arisen out of necessity to support individual research and/or clinical trials, which are often disease centered. The coexistence or development of a central biorepository can create varying degrees of conflict with existing satellite banks. It is important to work through the processes, principles, and values of the biorepositories before embarking on the idea of a central biorepository. Each system (satellite and central) has its pros and cons. The successful, cooperative management of both systems is best accomplished by having discussions with the stakeholders of each before making the final decision to implement a central biorepository.

The concept of a central biorepository has been advocated to allow for broad-scale collection, processing, storage, and distribution of normal and disease tissue for use in basic and translational research, as well as in support of clinical trials. With institutional support, such a central biorepository could offer significant advantages to investigators and clinicians, such as detailed pathology support and analysis of tissue, standardized quality control of tissue, adequately funded storage space that allows for backup freezers, and access for investigators to specimens from a broad array of tumor types. However, in many instances, such a centralized and robust infrastructure has been widely absent in most institutions. In these situations, investigators have developed their own directed satellite banks that have allowed for collection of necessary patient specimens and ensuring that appropriate consent has been obtained and that patients are followed up. In many instances, such satellite banks have required extensive investment by the investigator, including allocation of research funds and development of customized storage and databases that allow for information and specimen retrieval. It is therefore no surprise that owners of satellite banks may be wary of the inception of a central biorepository, thus leading to potential conflict.

There is no clearly defined way in which to readily merge existing satellite banks with a newly developed central biorepository (or even to determine if this should be undertaken). In many cases, satellite banks raise a number of variables regarding specimen collection and storage protocols, quality assessment of tissue specimens, and discrete database elements that may not be readily generalizable into a central network. Furthermore, the personal investment of research time and resources by the investigator gives rise to a sense of "ownership" over specimens that have been stored within such a satellite facility. Finally, performing a retroactive assessment of all satellite-bank–derived specimens that would include required quality elements set by a central biorepository may take up significant personnel time that can be better used for prospective specimen collection. Thus, in institutions that are developing a central biorepository, a cooperative relationship with existing satellite banks may be of value. Specifically, encouraging satellite banks to share existing tissue with interested investigators and encouraging satellite banks to utilize the central biorepository for future collections may be valuable to enhance tissue use, reduce costs, and maximize quality. Such an arrangement may allow the investigators who manage satellite banks to prospectively make use of new resources and facilities developed by a central biorepository, without losing control over specimens to which they have devoted significant financial and research time commitments.

Balancing Departmental Versus Institutional Needs for a Central Biorepository

A centralized biorepository has the potential to satisfy the needs of both the pathology department and the institution, with the caveats that adequate funding is assured for infrastructure and priorities for tissue use are established by general agreement. Methods by which to streamline agreements about specimen use include the establishment of an oversight board for the biorepository, a clear mission for the role of the central biorepository, involvement of stakeholders along disease-specific or organ-based lines, and a clear prioritization of specimen allocation and use. Such oversight and regulation have become increasingly important as the number of tissue and body fluid requests have increased to meet the needs of translational research and new drug development.

In general, there are three major uses of specimens that are stored in biorepositories. First, a primary role for the central biorepository is to facilitate clinical trials and/or therapeutics that are specifically designed to improve patient care. Such a role could potentially include tissue procurement to support ancillary studies as part of a national or multi-institutional clinical trial. Other such efforts might include gene sequencing for specific mutations related to clinical therapeutics or participation in efforts such as the Cooperative Human Tissue Network (CHTN, www.chtn.nci.nih.gov). Such endeavors promote the institutional mission of enhancing patient care and support the role of clinicians who are actively involved in clinical trials. Remuneration from such trials may be modest and should be directed specifically to the department housing the biospecimen repository to support such efforts.

A second goal of a central biorepository is to support internal investigators (either funded or nonfunded) who will use human specimens to further research discoveries. In this way, the biorepository will also facilitate the acquisition of external funding for future research. Publications and grants that arise from such an endeavor clearly enhance the academic prestige of the institution, which may attract patients seeking high-quality clinical treatment on the cutting edge of medical care.

A third goal of biorepository tissue use is to satisfy contracts between the institution and external entities, such as industry and tissue-marketing centers, thereby perhaps providing a useful source of revenue to subsidize future research and operational costs. This third arena of tissue use may be somewhat contentious, given that some rare specimen types may be leveraged for significant financial gain to the institution rather than for internal research purposes. In such instances, oversight by disease-specific stakeholders and the regulatory body of the biospecimen repository may be necessary to establish institutional priorities for rare tissue use.

Obtaining Institutional Support for Enforcement of Pathology-Based Biorepository Policies

Ideally, support for pathology-driven best practices and biospecimen collection should be obtained from the institutional leadership. It is clear that optimal tissue collection processes should be established within the pathology department, with the assistance of the pathologist, resident, and technicians who participate in the biorepository effort. Such processes may include determining the amount of tissue that can be spared for biobanking, oversight of gross descriptions of all specimens, and review of quality-control sections performed at the time of biospecimen collection. Institutional oversight is critical in both promoting awareness of standards of practice, as well as in enforcing new policies that are established by the biorepository. Furthermore, pathologists should become actively involved not only as technical experts, but also as advisors within disease-specific advisory groups or as members of the oversight board of the biorepository.

References

1. Dayal S, Murray J, Wilson K, Lannigan A. Imprint cytology from core biopsies increases the sensitivity of fine needle aspiration (FNA) in breast cancer patients. *Magy Seb.* 2011;64:59-62.
2. Liu A. Laser capture microdissection in the tissue biorepository. *J Biomol Tech.* 2010;21:120-125.
3. Finkelstein SD, Bibbo M, Loren DE, et al. Molecular analysis of centrifugation supernatant fluid from pancreaticobiliary duct samples can improve cancer detection. *Acta Cytol.* 2012;56:439-447.
4. Nurkka A, Obiero J, Käyhty H, Scott JA. Effects of sample collection and storage methods on antipneumococcal immunoglobulin A in saliva. *Clin Diagn Lab Immunol.* 2003;10:357-361.
5. Brambilla E, Strohmenger L, Vogel G. The effect of storage in liquid nitrogen on the isolation of oral yeasts in human saliva. *Arch Oral Biol.* 1992;37:237-239.
6. Assfalg M, Bertini I, Colangiuli D, et al. Evidence of different metabolic phenotypes in humans. *Proc Natl Acad Sci USA.* 2008;105:1420-1424.
7. Bertini I, Calabrò A, De Carli V, et al. The metabonomic signature of celiac disease. *J Proteome Res.* 2009;8:170-177.
8. Bernini P, Bertini I, Luchinat C, Nincheri P, Staderini S, Turano P. Standard operating procedures for pre-analytical handling of blood and urine for metabolomic studies and biobanks. *J Biomol NMR.* 2011;49:231-243.
9. Zhou H, Yuen PS, Pisitkun T, et al. Collection, storage, preservation, and normalization of human urinary exosomes for biomarker discovery. *Kidney Int.* 2006;69:1471-1476.

Chapter 3

Management and Key Personnel of the Biospecimen Repository

Nilsa C. Ramirez
Laura Monovich

Introduction

The primary objective of a biospecimen repository is the long-term acquisition, storage, processing, and disbursement of a large number of high-quality normal, diseased, and malignant biospecimens and related data (obtained with from proper consent from patients) for the purpose of supporting cutting-edge research. The biorepository should provide a full range of services for investigators involved in biospecimen research who wish to enhance their collection and research efforts. In order to support the base level of services and to optimize tissue-banking activities—such as specimen collection and processing, inventory management, universal electronic consent, and virtual microscopy review—the biorepository requires appropriate professional staffing and staff commitment.

Initially, many biorepositories were modeled after some of the usual areas found in hospital-based pathology laboratories, especially surgical pathology. This approach still works well for relatively small biorepositories that are based in pathology departments (usually supported by that infrastructure) and likely to be serving only institutional investigators. Standard operating procedures (SOPs) developed in the clinical laboratory setting (under the guidance of the Clinical Laboratory Improvement Amendments [CLIA] and the College of American Pathologists [CAP] Biorepository Accreditation Program) serve as templates for many SOPs used in biorepositories. These SOPs provide efficient methodologies already known to be associated with high-quality standards. However, as tissue procurement, storage, and testing evolve, these pathology-laboratory–based models don't necessarily support more complex operations. Larger biorepositories need more complex infrastructures that can accommodate the multiple demands of different types of investigators, different kinds of projects (from discovery phase studies to translational research), and interactions at various levels (from the host institution to multi-institutional collaborative efforts). Many biorepositories are also involved in sophisticated tissue processing and testing in order to assist investigators with limited resources, expedite time-sensitive studies, and provide high-quality testing in a cost-effective manner.

As the demand for biorepository services increases, many sponsors are looking for guidance as they develop their own facilities and try to customize biorepository services to fulfill their present and future needs. At this time, two comprehensive best-practices documents can assist in the development or updating of a biorepository. One document was originally published in 2005 by the International Society for Biological and Environmental Repositories (ISBER)[1] and is now in its second version; a third version should be available for publication in 2012. The other document is the 2011 updated version of the National Cancer Institute's *NCI Best Practices for Biospecimen Resources* (NCI Best Practices).[2] These two documents provide detailed narratives that can assist in the development of different areas of a biorepository in a manner that is not only structured and efficient, but is in compliance with national and international regulations that deal with a variety of laboratory settings and ethical issues related to human subjects' research and patient confidentially.

Organizational Structure of the Biospecimen Repository

To function efficiently, the biorepository must be organized in a manner consistent with its mission, as defined by the sponsoring institution(s) or group(s). Once the mission is established, the organizational structure should be developed, taking into consideration several factors, including (1) the physical facility and its location, (2) the resources available for biorepository development and continuous support, and (3) the types of activities expected from this resource by its sponsors (eg, community hospital, comprehensive cancer center, university medical center, NCI's Clinical Trials Cooperative Group Program, disease-specific advocacy group) and by the investigators whom it is designed to serve.

The physical facility occupied by the biorepository should have sufficient space to support its operation, including a biospecimen processing area and storage. Even when a biorepository has the most desirable physical facility, it still needs adequate staffing. To ensure high-quality biospecimens, the NCI Best Practices describes biospecimen resources personnel needs as follows[2]:

> Personnel involved in biospecimen resource management and use including researchers, technicians, nurses, surgeons, pathologists, anesthesiologists, and assistants are aware of the purpose and goals of the biospecimen resource (see Section B.1.2.1, Related Personnel Descriptions and Roles). To ensure the collection of high-quality biospecimens for research, personnel are well qualified and trained to adhere to applicable SOPs [standard operating procedures]. Update training of personnel should be conducted on a periodic basis, in accordance with applicable regulations and position descriptions (ISBER 2008). A pathologist or his/her designee—such as a pathology assistant or another individual with applicable training and judgment—should be involved in collecting and processing anatomic pathology biospecimens, including surgical and autopsy tissue and body fluids. It is important that a pathologist determines which biospecimen or portion thereof is necessary for complete evaluation and which is excess (remnant tissue) that may be provided to the biospecimen resource for research purposes. The involvement of a pathologist in this process is crucial in order to ensure that patient care is not compromised.

A relatively simple organizational structure composed of a director and a group of managers and/or coordinators who can identify and streamline the activities of the laboratory technician(s) in the biorepository will better serve a resource based in a single institution or at one physical facility. However, a multi-institutional consortium will need a more complex structure that can handle the needs of the independent units and their various responsibilities as well as a centralized organizational structure that can coordinate all the separate units in a coherent, cost-efficient, and time-efficient manner. The structure of the biorepository may have additional complexity, depending on the nature of the biobanking efforts of all or some of the multi-institutional units, including those that involve combinations of physical banks and virtual banks, and those that have off-site units with duplicated services as part of a disaster recovery strategy.

Resources available for the development and continuous support of the biorepository will determine how much to invest in personnel (salaries, benefits), physical facilities (space for future growth, freezer room, virtual microscopy setting, slide storage), and equipment (supplies, freezers), therefore affecting the organizational structure. A biorepository can be funded by a single source or by a combination of sources (eg, institutional and/or departmental funds, federal government and/or foundation grants) in response to institutional, regional, national, and/or international needs. A biorepository with a sizable budget can probably afford at least the part-time leadership services of a pathologist or a PhD-level scientist with expertise in biobanking, as well as the full- or part-time services of nurses, medical technologists, pathology assistants, specialized pathologists, and individuals well versed in medical information technologies. A more restrictive budget would likely limit the number of individuals involved in the operation as well as the time commitments of those with expertise in biobanking. It can also lead to the hiring of individuals with limited experience who are likely to need on-the-job training in the area of biobanking.

The types of activities expected from the biorepository by the sponsor(s) as well as by the investigators it is designed to serve will definitively impact the organizational structure by determining the type of training and the number of employees needed to run the facility. For example: a hospital-based biorepository can collect several malignant tissue samples from a patient to fulfill the requirements of patient enrollment in an ongoing institutional or NCI-sponsored cancer cooperative group clinical trial (and to bank for future research). The institution is likely to obtain consent from the patient for all of these uses at the time of admission. This duty should be performed by a trained medical professional (usually a nurse) who can work full- or part-time for that institution, depending on the volume of patients. However, a clinical trials cancer cooperative group biobank will receive the consented specimen from the affiliated institution but is not responsible for hiring and paying for the consenting institutional medical professional (although the cancer cooperative group biobank may be involved in the initial and/or ongoing training associated with informed consent).

Figure 3-1 is an example of the organizational structure of a freestanding large biorepository that handles at least 50,000 biospecimens per year; key personnel are described in the next section. It is important to remember that in many organizations the title assigned to a particular job may be determined by their human resources (HR) department on the basis of the level of administrative duties (as defined by the institution) and the pay scale, rather than being determined by the biorepository's "home" department

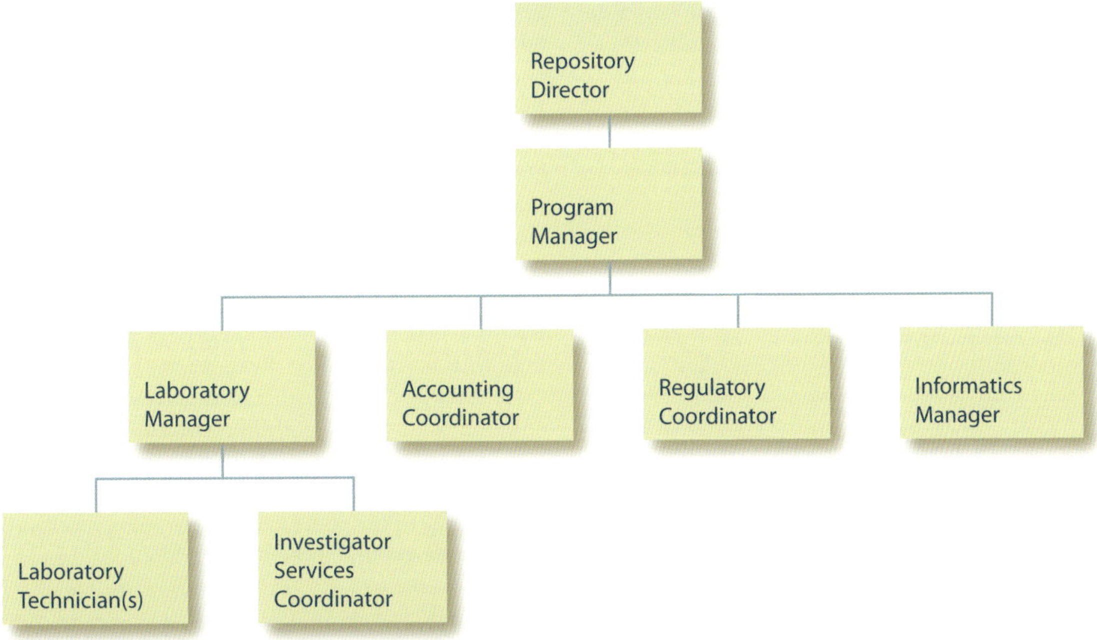

Figure 3-1. Biorepository organizational structure.

or division. It is possible that the title of "coordinator" in a particular institution is considered management level (usually a higher pay scale and numerous responsibilities), but in another institution it is not. Before assigning titles to your biorepository employees, check with your institutional HR department and clarify these designations so they match your expectations and your budget. You can use the recommended job descriptions listed below in association with the best title consistent with your expectations and your institution's qualifications and restrictions. You can also work with your HR department to create new positions and classifications (especially if you expect to hire more than one individual at the same level). The institution's HR department should guide you regarding comparable institutional salaries and benefits. Inquire at other institutions that have an established biorepository similar to the one you want to create or expand regarding employees' titles, salaries, benefits, and coverage (shifts).

The Biospecimen Repository Director

The biorepository Director should be a qualified professional with a medical degree or advanced graduate degree (MD, DO, PhD, ScD), with experience and knowledge of biorepository operations and activities, experience in clinical laboratory management, and knowledge of current regulations and procedures designed to protect human subjects in the context of biospecimen-based research. The Director is responsible for the administration and operation of biorepository activities, including oversight to ensure that the procurement, storage, processing, and distribution of biospecimens occurs without loss or waste of resources; that there is immediate and central data collection affiliated with the biospecimens; that SOPs are regularly updated (based on current biobanking guidelines and best practices, covering all aspects of biorepository activities); and that concept development includes consideration of all aspects of biospecimen collection, processing, and analysis. The Director is also responsible for the development and implementation of the organizational structure of the biorepository, including documenting staff responsibilities and overseeing and approving job descriptions. Along with the Program Manager, the Director ensures that there is appropriate staffing capable of performing repository activities and that the assigned duties are commensurate with their capabilities. Other roles of the Director include participation in the governance review process, biorepository budget preparation (including writing and managing grants to support some or all biorepository efforts, if applicable), determination of biospecimen adequacy (quality assurance [QA]/quality control [QC]), development of record-keeping policies compliant with current biobanking guidelines and best practices, and guidance in the use of proper methodology and new technologies. The Director is in charge of overseeing the fulfillment of the biorepository's mission statement and participates in activities as designated by the Governance Committee.

The ISBER *2012 Best Practices for Repositories* defines the biorepository Director's role as follows[1]:

> The Director should implement policies of the organization and should be responsible for all operations, including compliance with current national, state and local regulations. Depending upon organizational structure of the repository, the Director may have other responsibilities including: (i) ensuring that the repository operates within budget, (ii) ensuring that the repository has adequate funding for operations which may require the development of cost-recovery strategies to ensure the repository's short and long-term financial stability, (iii) ensuring that an adequate policy is in place for access to the specimens stored in the repository and that requests for specimens are met in a timely fashion, (iv) serving as a liaison to key users (v) ensuring confidentiality of data and (vi) ensuring that standard operating procedures (SOPs) and best practices are in place and in general use.

A pathologist with expertise in biobanking should be part of any biorepository, especially if the repository's Director is not a pathologist. In this setting, the degree of involvement of a pathologist should be defined by the repository's Director and the Governance or Oversight Committee (see below). A pathologist should complement the duties of the Director and cover issues such as tissue procurement techniques, biospecimen QA/QC, and histology-related issues. Several pathologists should be available to assist the Director if the workload increases, and at least one pathologist should participate in the Governance or Oversight Committee.

Key Personnel of the Biospecimen Repository

Program Manager

The Program Manager (or Program Director in some institutions) manages the day-to-day operations of the biorepository. The sole purpose of this position is to assist the Director in finding ways to make the biorepository more productive by providing effective methods in its business operations. The Program Manager will prepare program budgets, manage inventory, handle logistics, manage security issues, and assist in hiring and supervising employees. This individual should have experience and knowledge of biobanking activities, a strong leadership background, and must be able to handle problems quickly and efficiently. Additional responsibilities include (but are not limited to) managing process and performance improvement, planning and implementing operation strategies, and cost management. This position (with the Director's approval) will provide documentation of staff duties and responsibilities, maintain updated job descriptions, perform staff performance reviews, and develop and maintain training programs, ensuring that all federal, state, and local requirements are met. The Program Manager must have excellent oral and written communication skills, be highly organized, and have the ability to interact with all levels within the organization and with the investigators. Depending on the complexity of the operation, desirable qualifications include a master's degree in a scientific field or a bachelor's degree in medical technology or science, and 8 to 10 years of bench work experience in a similar laboratory setting. In a smaller biorepository setting, if this position is not necessary, some of the duties described under the Program Manager can be absorbed by the Laboratory Manager and some of the coordinators (see below), because they should respond directly to the biorepository Director.

Laboratory Manager

The Laboratory Manager is responsible for the day-to-day operation of the biorepository, including (but not limited to) the procurement, processing, storing, and distributing of specimens, as well as supervision and training of the laboratory's technicians. This position requires experience and knowledge in a research and/or clinical laboratory setting. The Laboratory Manager oversees the overall process of specimen collection and data entry, preparation and processing of tissue for testing (including QA/QC), biobanking, and distribution. This individual will work closely with the Director and Program Manager in the development, implementation, and maintenance of SOPs and policies. The position will assist in the execution of the training program and the overall quality assessment and assurance processes. The Laboratory Manager must have excellent oral and written communication skills, be highly organized, and have the ability to interact with all levels within the organization and with the investigators. Depending on the complexity of the operation, desirable qualifications include a bachelor's degree in medical technology or science and at least 5 years of bench work experience in a similar laboratory setting.

Informatics Manager

The Informatics Manager is responsible for the analysis, interface design, implementation planning, training, and frontline support of the repository informatics systems. This position also entails performance of analyses to confirm information accuracy, ensuring the proper collection and editing of required information. The experience and knowledge of the

Informatics Manager requires a strong information technology (IT) background with development and programming experience. This position assists in design specifications, data exchange, business negotiations, and ensuring ongoing support. The Informatics Manager will resolve issues throughout the repository's operational, management, business, marketing, and strategic planning needs. The Informatics Manager assists in staff activities related to the information systems activities (eg, assignment of staff, development of work plans, monitoring of system design and development progress, coordination of system training, implementation support, and ongoing system support and maintenance). The individual should coordinate and recommend system design specifications and business processes for all IT initiatives (including virtual microscopy and biospecimen inventory), as well as evaluate and make recommendations for improvements to current information systems. The Informatics Manager is responsible for the development and implementation of procedures related to information system activities. The individual should stay informed of trends, leading-edge technology, and developments in health care information systems and management by attending professional conferences, reading professional literature, and networking with colleagues at local, national, and international health care organizations. The Informatics Manager must have excellent oral and written communication skills, be highly organized, and have the ability to interact with all levels within the organization and with the investigators. Depending on the complexity of the operation, desirable qualifications include a bachelor's or master's degree in computer information systems, statistics/biostatistics, epidemiology, or other related field with a minimum of 3 to 5 years experience in a health care industry or life sciences as well as 2 years of previous management experience.

Accounting Coordinator

The Accounting Coordinator assists the Program Manager with the fiscal-related projects and daily duties that include (but are not limited to) ordering of equipment and supplies, invoicing of services rendered, and monitoring and maintaining financial activities. The Accounting Coordinator should work closely with the finance and grant staff of the institution. Additional responsibilities include addressing problems with vendors regarding quality of products and supplies (including getting equipment repaired and replaced); preparing and submitting reports to the biorepository Director and Program Manager monthly or as needed; contacting vendors, manufacturers, and distributors for price quotes; and assisting the Program Manager in maintaining fiscal records for grant maintenance, grant preparation, and reporting purposes. This individual should have knowledge of and experience with accounting practices. The Accounting Coordinator must have excellent oral and written communication skills, be highly organized, and have the ability to interact with all levels within the organization and with the investigators. Depending on the complexity of the operation, desirable qualifications include a bachelor's or master's degree in accounting or business administration with at least 5 years of experience in laboratory-related accounting practices. For those institutions funded by federal and/or foundation grants, at least 3 years of experience in research administration is recommended.

Regulatory Coordinator

The Regulatory Coordinator organizes and administers research-study–associated activities. This position assists in project planning and ensures that preestablished work scope, study protocol, and regulatory requirements are followed. This role, working closely with the Investigator Services Coordinator, includes obtaining documentation of Institutional Review Board (IRB) approval for all approved projects, preparation and maintenance of human subjects research project submissions to the IRB, documenting human research subjects protections education and training for all biorepository employees, and coordinating material transfer agreements with approved investigator's sites. The Regulatory Coordinator is responsible for developing, initiating, maintaining, and revising policies and procedures for the general operation of the biorepository compliance program and its related activities to prevent illegal, unethical, or improper conduct and to promote integrity and compliance throughout the biorepository. The Regulatory Coordinator recruits research subjects, as appropriate, and serves as principal administrative liaison for particular projects. In the proper setting, this person also obtains informed consent from patients for institution-based studies and biobanking efforts. Depending on the complexity of the operation, desirable qualifications include a background in health care (eg, nurse, physician's assistant, clinical research associate) and excellent oral and written communication skills.

Investigator Services Coordinator

The Investigator Services Coordinator is responsible for conducting a first-time review of all received applications for specimens to assure that the applications are complete and clear. This position works closely with the Program and Laboratory Managers to ensure that investigators' requests are reasonable. Communication with the investigators to negotiate a more reasonable request and/or to deal with logistics is performed by this position as well as any duties related to investigator services, including gathering and analyzing inventory and shipping data and providing reports as needed. The person must have excellent oral and written communication skills and be highly organized. Depending on the complexity of the operation, desirable qualifications include a background as a clinical and/or research laboratory technician or as a clinical research associate.

Laboratory Technician(s)

The Laboratory Technician will perform routine and semicomplex processing of biospecimens (solid and liquid) according to SOPs. This position is responsible for biospecimen procurement and processing (under proper supervision), biospecimen storage, biospecimen distribution, and for obtaining associated documents and data from—and providing them to—individual investigators, participating institutions, the reviewing pathologist, and collaborating laboratories. The Laboratory Technician is responsible for responding to various inquiries relating to repository activities, entering data into appropriate databases, and performing various laboratory techniques (eg, in the areas of cytology, hematology, and histology) and procedures. The Laboratory Technician should be fully qualified in biological laboratory techniques, with an understanding of histology, cytology, and nucleic acid and protein processing. Depending on the complexity of the operation, desirable qualifications include formal laboratory training and certification (if applicable) in the areas of surgical pathology (tissue procurement technician), hematology (medical technologist), and histology (histotechnician).

According to the ISBER *2012 Best Practices for Repositories,* the technical staff responsibilities are defined as follows[1]:

- Staff should possess sufficient educational background, experience, and training to assure that assigned tasks are performed in accordance with the repository's established SOPs.
- Technical staff should be responsible for adherence to policies and SOPs as established by the Director.
- Duties of each staff member should coincide with written job descriptions.
- Staff should demonstrate competency in operations for which they have received training and to which they are assigned.
- Authority and reporting relationships for each member of the staff should be clearly described.

If the biorepository is small, it is not uncommon to use other institutional resources for the performance of complex laboratory procedures in areas of histology, nucleic acid extractions, cell culture, and protein handling. In this setting, the tests can be performed by specialized core facilities or clinical laboratory services.

Staff Training Requirements

Staff training is a necessary requirement for all repository personnel. Training should include (but is not limited to) biohazards (ie, bloodborne pathogens) and chemical hazards. The more complex processes of the biorepository may subject its staff to different training needs. Safety training should be completed before the start of any "hands-on" activity involving safety hazards. Other types of training that should be covered include privacy protection and confidentiality issues (informed consent and the Health Insurance Portability and Accountability Act of 1996 [HIPAA] Privacy Rule) and any institutional, local, state, or federal regulatory requirements for laboratory personnel. In the biorepository setting, it is also important to familiarize the staff with the commonly used "honest broker" model (where the biorepository is considered to be neutral and able to mediate between two parties—usually the tissue source site and the investigator—as the custodian of the biospecimen, protecting the patient's privacy without compromising the patient's confidentiality).

Currently, no specific certification requirements exist for personnel working exclusively in biorepositories (although many professionals routinely employed in a biorepository may be certified in various fields, including laboratory medicine and information technologies). However, a minimum level of experience and knowledge in laboratory procedures and in handling of human biospecimens is required. Biorepositories housed at institutions (eg, hospitals, universities, or research centers) have to follow institutional policies regarding safety and handling of hazardous material. All repository personnel, including non-laboratory staff, should be trained in safety regarding the hazards with which individuals may come into contact while working within the biorepository space. Repository staff is responsible for protecting non-laboratory staff by ensuring that laboratory areas are secured to prevent unauthorized entry and that hazards are appropriately labeled. Some portions of the biorepository may be involved in patient care in a manner that requires specific personnel training and laboratory procedure certification by appropriate accrediting bodies (eg, CAP).

Biorepository staff training should be job, task, and location specific. The extent of the training should match the operational needs of the tasks and areas of work. Training should involve instruction and sign-off in the use of any equipment that employees are asked to use. The level of training must be appropriate to the employee's level of comprehension. Training tools may include (but are not limited to) any combination of reviewing written procedures, participating in web-based training sessions, viewing training videos, observing other personnel, and direct hands-on training. Records of critical completed elements of training should be maintained. Appropriate training elements to be documented may include attendance at specific training sessions (especially those related to safety), review of key SOPs, completion of any tests or certifications, and trainer evaluation of key tasks. A record should be maintained of when the employee reviewed key procedures or, preferably, demonstrated competency in the performance of each key procedure. Any employee feedback relevant to an SOP should be provided to the appropriate supervisor to facilitate periodic review and revisions of SOPs. To ensure consistency in the performance of repository activities, training should also be monitored as part of the QA program, including a review by supervisors, on a regular basis, of practices and performance of certain tasks to assure that they are being executed in accordance with the SOPs.

Training Resources

- Office for Human Research Protections (OHRP): http://www.hhs.gov/ohrp
- International Air Transport Association (IATA): http://www.iata.org/training
- Good Laboratory and Manufacturing Practices: http://www.qualityassociatesinc.com/
- International Civil Aviation Organization (ICAO): http://www.icao.int/Pages/default.aspx
- Collaborative Institutional Training Initiative (CITI): https://www.citiprogram.org/Default.asp
- Protecting Human Research Participants: http://phrp.nihtraining.com/users/login.php
- Good Clinical Practice: http://www.fda.gov/ScienceResearch/SpecialTopics/RunningClinicalTrials/default.htm
- ISBER Best Practices for Repositories: http://www.isber.org

Training Responsibilities

Responsibility for training and documentation of training may vary from institutional and divisional requirements. The biorepository Director should ensure that appropriate training is provided to all staff members, key elements of training are documented, and local SOPs are maintained and updated according to biorepository guidelines. The biorepository Director or designee(s) should closely coordinate issues related to training in safety with the organization's Safety Office and with other individuals responsible for specific areas of repository procedures (eg, shipping and handling).

Any individual providing training for biorepository staff should have demonstrated training in and knowledge of the tasks for which they will be providing instruction. In addition to local SOPs, they should be aware of general repository policies for the area in which they are providing instruction. The trainer is responsible for assuring that the trainee understands each procedure and task fully. Successful performance of the task should be observed and documented by the trainer. For special areas of training (eg, human subjects protection, privacy, and safety), personnel or agencies with special expertise may provide the training, which is frequently web based. Online training permits employees to complete special areas of training at their own pace.

During the training period, the trainer should demonstrate, explain, and review the standards to be followed in conducting the procedure(s). The trainer should supervise the trainee in all tasks of the procedure(s) and provide feedback on the trainee's performance. Any employee performing a new task should be closely monitored until the task is performed proficiently. Supplemental training should be provided as needed.

Training Documentation

As training is completed, either for each individual task or for an entire area, a record of training completion should be made. This documentation may include the names of trainers/trainees and training sessions, test results, SOP titles and dates, certifications received, etc, as appropriate. Requirements for documentation of training may differ among biorepositories, depending upon institutional and regulatory requirements. At a minimum, documentation of training should be maintained by the biorepository for each staff member. Some permanent training records may be maintained by other departments of the institution, as per local requirements. The training record may be part of the personnel file. Documentation should include the following:

- Copies of any certification of specialized training of the employee, especially in the areas of shipping, safety, and pertinent governmental regulations, including training mandated by a regulatory agency or the sponsoring institution, the local IRB, and the privacy board (HIPAA); Occupational Safety and Health Administration (OSHA)-required training in safety; and training in shipping
- Documentation that an employee has been provided with all SOPs pertinent to the employee's responsibilities

The employees' training records should be kept in the repository administration office and be available for QA review. The training file may be archived according to the institutional requirements after the employee is separated from the organization. If employees move from the repository to other departments within the institution, employees should be allowed to take copies of their training records with them.

Training Frequency

Training should be conducted in accordance with federal, state, and local regulations and also as needed for new staff, new equipment, and any new tasks. Training typically occurs at the start of employment and annually thereafter (eg, biohazard and chemical hazard training, issues related to the IRB and HIPAA, and IATA shipping). Training for critical areas should be performed according to a defined schedule. Supplemental training should be provided as needed—whenever deficiencies are noted in either individual or team performance or when changes in SOPs are made to improve future performance or to prevent recurrence of undesirable outcomes.

Continuing Scientific Education

Continuing scientific education is offered by many groups and institutions (eg, professional organizations, accrediting agencies, and vendors/manufacturers). Professional organizations in the areas of pathology (eg, the CAP, American Society for Clinical Pathology [ASCP], United States and Canadian Academy of Pathology [USCAP]), oncology/research (eg, American Association for Cancer Research [AACR], American Society of Clinical Oncology [ASCO]), and biobanking (eg, ISBER) already offer regular educational opportunities that appeal to biorepository-based personnel. General expansion of job knowledge and ongoing education may include training by senior staff, guest lectures, departmental training, and other opportunities that may enhance job satisfaction and performance.

Time and Salary Commitment

The biorepository and its leadership must consider and identify the following: personnel who will perform the tasks, funding to support the tasks described, necessary equipment, and space to perform the relevant activities. Salaries are usually the biggest expense in the biorepository budget. In a large, complex biorepository, the salary component of the budget can be considerable if there is a need for full-time, highly educated personnel. Funding estimates should include costs reflecting the time required for a staff member to collect and process biospecimens, considering all steps of the various processing routines: retrieval from storage and packaging the samples, as well as retrieval of existing accompanying paperwork. Equipment purchases and maintenance agreements must also be taken into account. In some settings, investigators obtain specimens free of charge, because the cost associated with specimen collection, banking, processing, and distribution is covered by the sponsoring institution or group; however, in other settings, there is a structured specimen "fee for service," paid by the investigator, that generates program income. Depending on the budget, the program income can be used to cover miscellaneous expenses (eg, travel to conferences, equipment upgrades), salaries, and/or supplies.

The time that employees (full-time and part-time) should devote to biorepository-related activities will be determined by the size of the operation and the complexity of each task. The biorepository Director should determine the need for each employee and the level of involvement in any particular task. Although a basic organizational structure should be in place in order to comply with the mission of the biorepository, enough flexibility should exist to allow the system to introduce additional employees (part time, contingent, or full time) if needed. Salaries are usually determined by the host institution's HR department and are influenced by the geographical location of the host institution. In some settings, salary limitations are complemented by bonuses (eg, based on productivity, seniority) or other long-term incentives (eg, additional vacation days, book and/or travel funds, tuition reimbursement).

Interactions With the Institutional Review Board

The interactions between a biorepository and the investigators it serves are regulated in order to avoid legal and ethical issues that could interfere with the proper utilization of human specimens for research. The Institutional Review Board/Ethics Review Committee (IRB/ERC) evaluates research involving human subjects at an institutional level. Part of the job of the IRB/ERC is the assessment of the SOPs and processes designed by the biorepository for the purpose of acquiring, storing, processing, and disbursing biospecimens to approved investigators. Therefore, upon establishing a biorepository, evaluation by the IRB/ERC (of the institution that houses the biorepository) is required in order to allow it to function at full capacity. If the setting is that of a consortium of multiple institutions housing various components of a shared biorepository, each component needs to be evaluated by the IRB/ERC of each host institution. In this case, a centralized office will probably be needed to keep track of the IRB certificates for the consortium.

Once the biorepository is functional, it is expected to obtain a copy of any IRB/ERC-approved project submitted by each investigator before releasing any specimens for that particular project (this IRB/ERC approval process should cover the issue of informed consent for a particular project). Any future modification to a study that requires IRB/ERC approval should be communicated to the biorepository, and a copy of the updated document filed with the approved project documentation for future reference. If a study is exempt from IRB/ERC approval, it is common practice to obtain a document from an IRB/ERC officer (usually the chairperson of the IRB/ERC) indicating that the study does not meet the definition of "human subjects research" and that no further IRB review is needed. That document also should be filed by the biorepository with the approved project documentation from that investigator for future reference.

If a biorepository is involved with international projects, there should be a clear understanding of the rules and regulations of each foreign institution that is participating in any given project, regardless of the type of transaction (ie, foreign specimens being banked in the United States or US specimens being forwarded to investigators overseas). The biorepository should facilitate these transactions in a manner that is respectful of all national and international sensitivities (social and ethnic), protective of the privacy and confidentiality of the patients, and compliant with the laws of all countries involved. Several documents that deal with ethical issues in human subjects research can also assist a biorepository that is new to this type of international relationship—for example, the *WMA Declaration of Helsinki*[3] and *The Belmont Report*.[4]

Governance and Oversight

It is recommended that all biorepositories form a Governance Committee or Institutional Oversight Committee. The Governance Committee functions to review the use of the biorepository's services as well as the distribution of tissue from the biorepository. The goal of this governing body is to focus on providing the infrastructure and resources to support and facilitate basic science and translational research, ensuring tissue sources are used effectively and eliminating conflicts of interest. Formal interactions between the biorepository and outside institutions, organizations, vendors, and/or groups should also be monitored by the Institutional Oversight Committee, including evaluation of any type of contractual relationship in which the biorepository is involved. Plans to deal with large-scale tissue acquisition (eg, donations from another biorepository [legacy specimens], tissue donations by advocacy organizations, merging biorepositories) and the final disposition of the biospecimens if the biorepository closes operations should also be defined by this committee.

For a pathology-department–based biorepository, the Oversight Committee should be composed of at least four pathology department members actively involved in both service and research efforts (permanent members) and one clinician (ad hoc member). At least one member of the departmental administration (if possible, the director of surgical pathology or an equivalent) should be part of the Oversight Committee. Other representatives should include the biorepository Director and any active departmental investigator involved in basic research or translational research. Ad hoc clinician members can be chosen on the basis of expertise and should be contacted when their expert opinion is needed regarding a specific project. In this setting, the applications for biospecimens are usually to support small projects (mainly discovery phase studies). The Oversight Committee should meet at least twice a year to evaluate the status of the biorepository and more often, as needed, to evaluate the applications submitted by institutional investigators. Application approval should be based on the scientific value of the project, and initial feedback to the investigator regarding a project should take place in a timely manner (no more than 2 weeks after submission of the application).

If the biorepository is sponsored by an institution or group, the membership of the Oversight Committee should include institution/group leadership (senior administrative managers), pathologists, clinicians (including surgeons), basic and translational research scientists, a clinical data coordinator, select-

Table 3-1. Governance of a Biospecimen Repository

Title	Role	Members*
Biospecimen Repository	■ Receive, bank, inventory, and distribute specimens ■ Establish and monitor quality control and quality assurance standards and procedures ■ Promote repository resources and services ■ Establish an informatics resource	Biospecimen repository Director and staff
Utilization Committee	■ Provide oversight for the repository ■ Develop and upgrade policies to enhance specimen banking, quality, and distribution ■ Prioritize and support specimen banking and distribution ■ Ensure specimen availability to support basic science and translational research	Basic scientists, clinicians, and biorepository staff (Director and Program Manager)
Oversight Committee	■ Provide oversight for the repository and for the Utilization Committee ■ Direct basic science and translational research efforts ■ Develop and conduct clinical protocols and projects with basic science and translational research objectives, and publish results from these studies	Institutional/group leadership, and multidisciplinary advisory board members

* Overlapping membership of all three entities is expected in order to ensure continuity of information flow, policies, and procedures for enhancing productivity, efficiency, and resource management to prioritize and support projects and initiatives.

ed members of the Utilization Committee (see Table 3-1), nursing representatives (especially a research nurse), and a community patient advocate to ensure that issues concerning specimen availability, collection, quality, and utility can all be addressed.

A second committee (the Utilization Committee or Tissue Utilization Committee) assists the Governance or Institutional Oversight Committee in running the biorepository. The Utilization Committee consists of the biorepository Director and Program Manager, institutional scientists, and clinicians; its aim is to oversee the release of biospecimens on the basis of scientific merit, availability, and funding. Additional roles of the Utilization Committee are to guide the biorepository in its scientific and philosophical approach to tissue procurement and to facilitate any changes in biorepository operations with the Oversight Committee. The Utilization Committee, with input from the Oversight Committee, is responsible for developing and implementing the policies for the biorepository operations, including the development of a comprehensive biorepository application form for requesting biospecimens and any other biorepository-related services.

An application for use of biospecimens, documentation of an investigator's detailed research plan (with preliminary data, if available), any funding available for the project, and demonstration of local IRB approval are required for review by the Utilization Committee. Also required is the signed Material Use Agreement (MUA) or Material Transfer Agreement (MTA). The MUA/MTA limits the investigator's use of tissue for research purposes. This document represents an agreement between two organizations (the one that houses the biorepository and the investigator's institution) to transfer the biospecimens and the associated data, delineating their rights and responsibilities associated with a particular project. For an example of an MUA, please see Appendix at the end of this chapter (MUA developed by the National Cancer Institute's Group Banking Committee). All applications are reviewed for scientific merit and feasibility. New applications for biospecimens should be reviewed at least monthly.

To assist in the evaluation of the scientific merit of a project, the NCI Group Banking Committee developed the following criteria as a guideline (http://cgb.cancer.gov):

- Proven experience with the method proposed
- Standardized, validated, research biomarker assay methodology
- Research plan and budget appropriate to answer the study question
- Plan to compensate biorepository for provision of specimens (fee for service), if applicable
- Statistical design that shows that the study question can be addressed with the samples available
- Investigator has defined funding or proposal for funding submitted that is IRB submitted or approved

- Significance of study justifies use of tissue resource

The requested biospecimens from the biorepository can be made available to investigators after the application is approved and all required documents (MUA and IRB approval or documentation of exempted status) are forwarded to the biorepository. The Program Manager or Investigator Services Coordinator will inform the investigator of the approval/disapproval status of the project. Recommendations by the reviewers may become available to the applying investigator at this time.

Proper management of the biospecimen inventory is crucial to the mission of any biorepository. Specimen availability to investigators may be limited by several factors, including the number of required samples, the desired sample size, the presence of a specific amount of tumor/lesion tissue in each sample, and the presence/absence of necrosis. Although most consented samples usually remain in the biorepository until depletion, several circumstances may affect sample availability. For example, a patient may withdraw consent for biobanking at any time; if this occurs, all biospecimens from that patient must be destroyed. Upon receiving such written notification from the patient, the Program Manager is responsible for notifying the biorepository staff of the request to discard all specimens from a particular patient. Once the biospecimens in question are identified, the biorepository Director will authorize the destruction of the biospecimens in writing. The written documentation will be kept in the biorepository (in the patient's file) for future reference. Policies should also be in place to deal with different patient requests. Examples of these unusual circumstances include forwarding the banked biospecimens to (1) investigators not affiliated with the study the tissue was originally consented for, (2) a different clinical facility for patient-care–related testing, and (3) attorneys for litigation-related testing.

References

1. International Society for Biological and Environmental Repositories (ISBER). 2012 best practices for repositories: collection, storage, retrieval and distribution of biological materials for research. *Biopreserv Biobank.* 2012:10(2):79-161. Also available at www.isber.org. Accessed March 31, 2014.
2. Office of Biorepositories and Biospecimen Research, National Cancer Institute. *NCI Best Practices for Biospecimen Resources.* Washington, DC: National Institutes of Health, US Department of Health and Human Services; 2011. http://biospecimens.cancer.gov/practices/2011bp.asp. Accessed March 31, 2014.
3. World Medical Association. *WMA Declaration of Helsinki – Ethical Principles for Medical Research Involving Human Subjects.* Adopted by the 18th WMA General Assembly, Helsinki, Finland, June 1964, and amended by the: 29th WMA General Assembly, Tokyo, Japan, October 1975; 35th WMA General Assembly, Venice, Italy, October 1983; 41st WMA General Assembly, Hong Kong, September 1989; 48th WMA General Assembly, Somerset West, South Africa, October 1996; 52nd WMA General Assembly, Edinburgh, Scotland, October 2000; 53rd WMA General Assembly, Washington, DC, USA, October 2002 (Note of Clarification on paragraph 29 added); 55th WMA General Assembly, Tokyo, Japan, October 2004 (Note of Clarification on paragraph 30 added); 59th WMA General Assembly, Seoul, Korea, October 2008. http://www.wma.net/en/30publications/10policies/b3/index.html. Accessed March 31, 2014.
4. National Commission for the Protection of Human Subjects of Biomedical and Behavioral Research. *The Belmont Report. Ethical Principles and Guidelines for the Protection of Human Subjects of Research.* Washington, DC: National Institutes of Health, Department of Health, Education, and Welfare, Office of Human Subjects Research; April 18, 1979. http://www.hhs.gov/ohrp/humansubjects/guidance/belmont.html. Accessed March 31, 2014.

Appendix

MATERIAL USE AGREEMENT

Term – "Cooperative Group" used throughout this document includes the following organizations; The Alliance (ACOSOG, CALGB & NCCTG), COG, ECOG, NRG (NSABP, RTOG & GOG), SWOG and NCIC CTG.

(Cooperative Group), henceforth known as "PROVIDER" is pleased to be able to provide samples or derivatives thereof, ("MATERIAL") specified in Exhibit A, a research project proposal reviewed and approved by PROVIDER (incorporated by reference and hereinafter referred to as "RESEARCH", to Investigator at ______________________________ [Institution] (collectively "RECIPIENT"). PROVIDER is interested in supporting the research described in Exhibit A using the MATERIAL and will provide you with the MATERIAL subject to the following conditions on RECIPIENT's use of the MATERIAL. The conditions described below are necessary to insure that the MATERIAL is used solely for research and that PROVIDER's and RECIPIENT's interests in any possible commercialization of the product of research performed on the MATERIAL are protected.

Explanation of the Agreement

This agreement outlines the responsibilities and expectations of the listed RECIPIENT and PROVIDER. By signing the document RECIPIENT agrees to all terms and conditions defined below and understands that PROVIDER will uphold and enforce all terms and conditions outlined in the agreement, in accordance with Cooperative Group policy, upon release of any MATERIALS to RECIPIENT.

1. Scope of Work

MATERIAL is furnished to RECIPIENT for the purpose of the RESEARCH defined in Exhibit A and approved by appropriate scientific review committee defined by PROVIDER. Scope and nature of RESEARCH must be limited to that described in Exhibit A unless amended and approved by RECIPIENT and PROVIDER.

2. Funding

All aspects of the RESEARCH must be financially supported.

a. RECIPIENT agrees to arrange for payment of all additional charges associated with the processing and distribution of MATERIALS from the biorepository according to charge table provided to RECIPIENT (if applicable).
b. Documentation that the project has financial support must be furnished, signed by RECIPIENT's financial office, [Institutional Official] and must be provided to PROVIDER prior to RESEARCH activation and MATERIAL distribution.

If financial support is discontinued during the course of the study and alternative funding is not secured all research specimens and derivative samples will be returned to the respective biorepository, as specified herein under section entitled 'Termination of Agreement."

3. Safety of Personnel

RECIPIENT assumes all responsibility for informing and training personnel in the dangers and procedures for safe handling of human biospecimens and biohazards. All biorepository personnel must abide by OSHA regulations' pertaining to the handling of human specimens. RECIPIENT acknowledges awareness of and required compliance with OSHA regulations and will instruct staff to abide by these rules.

4. Stewardship of Material

All MATERIAL provided to RECIPIENT remains subject to PROVIDER'S stewardship and management. The Chairs of the Cooperative Groups agree that if samples are housed in more than one Cooperative Group, transfer of those samples to the PROVIDER or lead Cooperative Group repository will take place independently from this agreement.

5. Transfer of Material

a. The MATERIAL may not be assigned or sold to any other parties.
b. The MATERIAL may not be transferred by RECIPIENT to a third party/collaborator without first having obtained written approval of the transfer from PROVIDER. All such approved transfers must be accompanied by an agreement between RECIPIENT and the third party. The RECIPIENT is responsible for third party/collaborator to understand and abide by this agreement.
c. If the MATERIAL was obtained in connection with a study using a proprietary agent (ie, device or drug in additional to the human specimen) PROVIDER will refer to specific agreements or contingencies during review of RESEARCH proposal so that RECIPIENT may obtain a written agreement from the PROVIDER to perform the stated RESEARCH on the MATERIAL.
d. Both parties shall comply with all applicable laws and regulations, as amended from time to time, with respect to the collection, use, storage and disclosure of the MATERIAL and any related data, including without limitation, the Health Insurance Portability and Accountability Act of 1996 (HIPAA), its implementing regulations (45 CFR et seq) and the Common Rule (45 CFR 46)
e. RECIPIENT acknowledges that the conditions for use of MATERIAL are governed by Institutional Review Board (IRB) in accordance with Department of Health and Human Services regulations at 45 CFR 46. RECIPIENT agrees to comply fully with all such conditions and to report promptly to PROVIDER any proposed changes in RESEARCH and any unanticipated problems involving risks to subjects or others. RECIPIENT remains subject to applicable state or local laws or regulations and institution policies, which provide additional protections for human subjects. The MATERIAL may only be utilized in accordance with the conditions stipulated by IRB. Any additional use of MATERIAL beyond the RESEARCH requires prior review and approval by the PROVIDER, and, where appropriate, by an IRB at the RECIPIENT site, which must be convened under an applicable OHRP-approved Assurance.
f. RECIPIENT acknowledges that PROVIDER will not provide any information through which RECIPIENT may directly or indirectly identify the human subjects from whom the transferred Materials and/or data were obtained. RECIPIENT agrees not to seek such identifying information or attempt to identify subjects by any other means. If identifying information is received, RECIPIENT must notify PROVIDER immediately. RECIPIENT must promptly return the identifying information and/or MATERIAL as instructed by PROVIDER.

6. Use of Material

a. Use of the MATERIAL must be the RESEARCH and in compliance with any applicable laws and regulations governing the RECIPIENTS jurisdiction.
b. The MATERIAL must not be used in human subjects, in clinical trials, for diagnostic purposes involving human subjects, or to make any derivatives or progeny, as applicable, thereof without the written consent of PROVIDER.

c. With respect to any invention or discovery arising from the RESEARCH, the PROVIDER shall have an option to license to practice the invention or have it practiced for or on the PROVIDER's behalf with terms to be determined, as consistent with the NCI Cooperative Group agreement and Cooperative Group Guidelines.

7. Satellite Repository Responsibility of RECIPIENT

Any MATERIAL obtained as part of the RESEARCH are collected under the auspices and guidelines of PROVIDER whether or not the specimen is stored in the main repository or the RECIPIENT's laboratory. As such, all specimens and their derivatives are considered property of PROVIDER and remain under the stewardship of PROVIDER. RECIPIENT facility will serve as the interim repository for those specimens for the duration of the RESEARCH or until requested for return to PROVIDER's repository.

8. Data Submission and Analysis

a. Data analysis on data generated from RECIPIENT will be done by PROVIDER's statistical center or under their direction, according to design and analysis considerations agreed upon at the initiation of the project. All data must be submitted in the appropriate pre-approved format.
b. Availability of data generated in Cooperative Group studies will be in compliance with NIH and NCI data sharing policies and with Cooperative Group procedures.

9. Intellectual Property

The policy of the PROVIDER governing **intellectual property** rights continues through this agreement. This policy is based on PROVIDER's Cooperative agreement with the NCI and NCI Cooperative Group Guidelines and is available for review at http://ctep.cancer.gov/industryCollaborations2/intellectual_property.htm.

10. Publication

PROVIDER must be acknowledged in all abstracts and manuscripts, following guidelines agreed upon at the initiation of the specific project. All publications shall be submitted to PROVIDER for review and comment sixty (60) days prior to publication.

11. Confidentiality

a. In general, RECIPIENT will utilize only coded specimens and data and will not have access to the link to identify individuals who have contributed specimens. RECIPIENT agrees to maintain the confidentiality of all data and not to seek access to the link or seek any method to identify study subjects. Patient contact is forbidden for any reason, except in cases of specific IRB approval for specific protocol conditions and as approved by PROVIDER.
b. This agreement sets forth the terms and conditions pursuant to which PROVIDER may disclose certain Protected Health Information (PHI) to RECIPIENT. PHI may include associated demographic and clinical data that have been rendered a Limited Data set in compliance with 45 CFR 164.514(e)(1).
c. RECIPIENT ensures that any collaborator, as approved in writing by PROVIDER, working with RECIPIENT will agree to the same restrictions and conditions in writing that apply throughout this agreement.

12. Conflict of Interest

It is assumed that conflict of interest issues are dealt with internally by RECIPIENT, according to institutional policies. Investigator agrees by his/her signature and date on this agreement that such an institutional process has been followed and that no conflict of interest exists.

13. Termination of Agreement

a. Agreement will terminate upon conclusion of research to be performed using the Materials, or as a result of just cause upon request by PROVIDER. RECIPIENT agrees to discontinue use of the MATERIAL and will arrange for the return to PROVIDER, or its agent, or for the lawful disposal of all unused MATERIAL, as elected by PROVIDER.
b. This agreement may be terminated by PROVIDER upon five (5) days written notice to RECIPIENT if RECIPIENT breaches any provision contained in this agreement and such breach is not remedied within the five (5) day period. If such remedy is provided, proof of remedy will be required within the five (5) day period. Non-cause termination may be invoked by the PROVIDER, in certain cases.

14. Damage Waiver

a. MATERIAL is provided as a service to the research community without warranty, express or implied. PROVIDER assumes no responsibility for any injury (including death, damages, or loss) that may arise either directly or indirectly from their use. RECIPIENT agrees to assume all risks and responsibilities in connection with the receipt, handling, storage and use of MATERIAL.
b. Any material delivered pursuant to this agreement is understood to be experimental in nature and may have hazardous properties. Any material provided is provided as is and PROVIDER makes none and hereby disclaims all representations of warranties of any kind, either expressed or implied. There are no express or implied warranties of merchantability or fitness for a particular purpose, or that the use of the material will not infringe any patent, copyright, trademark or other proprietary rights.
c. **FOR STATE INSTITUTIONS:** RECIPIENT agrees to be responsible for any claims, costs, damages, or expenses resulting from any injury (including death), damage or loss that may arise solely from the receipt, handling, storage and use of biospecimens received from PROVIDER to the extent permitted under the laws of this State.
d. **FOR US GOVERNMENT AGENCIES:** On behalf of the United States Government, RECIPIENT assumes all risks and responsibilities in connection with the receipt, handling, storage and use of biospecimens received from PROVIDER. The United States assumes liability for any claims, damages, injury or expense arising from the use of the material or any derivative, but only to the extent provided under the Federal Tort Claims Act (28 USC Chap 171).
e. **FOR ALL OTHER INSTITUTIONS:** RECIPIENT agrees to assume all risks and responsibility in connection with the receipt, handling, storage and use of biospecimens. RECIPIENT agrees to defend, indemnify and hold PROVIDER and its directors, trustees, employees, agents harmless from any claims, liabilities, damages and losses that might arise as a result of RECIPIENT'S use of the MATERIALS.

15. Use of Name

Neither party shall use the names or trademarks of the other party or of any of the other party's affiliated entities in any advertising, publicity, endorsement, or promotion unless the other party has provided prior written consent for the particular use contemplated. The terms of this section survive the termination, expiration, non-renewal, or rescission of this Agreement.

16. Signatory Requirements

a. The undersigned warrant that they have authority to execute this agreement on behalf of the recipient institution.
b. This agreement constitutes the final, complete and exclusive agreement between the parties with respect to its subject matter and supersedes all past and contemporaneous

agreements, promises, and understandings, whether oral or written, between the parties. This agreement shall be binding upon and inure to the benefit of the parties, their heirs, legal representatives, successors and assigns. This agreement may not be amended or modified except by a writing signed by both parties and identified as an amendment to this agreement. Neither this agreement nor any of the rights or obligations under the agreement may be assigned by RECIPIENT without the written consent of PROVIDER. The failure of PROVIDER to insist at any time upon the strict observance or performance of any of the provisions of this agreement, or to exercise any right or remedy as provided in this agreement, will not impair any such right or remedy and will not be construed to be a waiver or relinquishment of the right or remedy. Execution of this agreement can be effected by facsimile signatures.

c. If you agree to these conditions, please sign in the space provided below as RECIPIENT Investigator and have an authorized representative of your Institution sign it also. The authorized representative should have authority over all investigators who might need access to the MATERIAL according to the terms of the research defined in Exhibit A.
d. Return the original signed copy of the agreement to:

   [insert PROVIDER address]:

   ____

   ____

   ____

ACCEPTED AND AGREED

The undersigned expressly certify or affirm that the contents of any statements made or reflected in this document are truthful and accurate. The undersigned further agree to examine and consider the subject matter of the Confidential Information on the foregoing basis.

FOR PROVIDER
Administrative Executive, Authorized Signatory

____
Printed Name

____
Title of Signatory

____
Signature

____
Date

Address:

____

____

FOR PROVIDER
Scientific/Medical Oversight, Authorized Signatory

____
Printed Name

____
Title of Signatory

____
Signature

____
Date

Address:

____

____

FOR RECIPIENT INSTITUTION, Authorized Signatory

____
Printed Name

____
Title of Signatory

____
Signature

____
Date

Address:

____

____

RECIPIENT INVESTIGATOR, Authorized Signatory

____
Printed Name

____
Title of Signatory

____
Signature

____
Date

Address:

____

____

Chapter 4

Infrastructure of the Biospecimen Repository and Associated Core Laboratories

M. Scott Lucia
Adrie van Bokhoven

Historically, many so-called "biobanking" efforts to collect patient samples were performed ad hoc by individual clinician scientists whose primary interest was to analyze the samples for specific scientific questions related to their own research purposes. Maintenance of sample residuals for future use became a byproduct of the research. This practice, while perhaps necessary at the time, resulted in quantities of isolated banks of specimens that were collected and handled using a wide range of methods of variable rigor, which limited the utility for research beyond the original intended studies.[1] Often such banks were housed in freezer units within a specific researcher's laboratory and not publicly advertised or made available.

Because the practice of obtaining specimens and conducting research, particularly genetic research, on patients' samples was becoming complicated by changes in regulations—such as the Health Insurance Portability and Accountability Act of 1996 (HIPAA) and the US Food and Drug Administration (FDA) human subjects protection regulations—and patient/community concerns regarding such research, the National Cancer Advisory Board conducted a study of 125 National Cancer Institute (NCI)-supported biorepositories to inventory their quality, practice patterns, and effectiveness.[1] The study showed lack of (1) standardized or optimal methods and management of biospecimens, (2) computerized informatics using common definitions, (3) responsiveness to the needs of researchers, and (4) legal and ethical policies. To address these findings, the NCI Office of Biorepositories and Biospecimen Research (now Biorepositories and Biospecimen Research Branch) organized two workshops in 2005 that brought together representatives from the biorepository, cancer, ethics, and informatics communities to propose approaches to unify and standardize biospecimen collection, management, handling, annotation, and distribution policies and procedures. From this came the development of the *First-Generation Guidelines for NCI-Supported Biorepositories*[2] as a first step toward defining standardized best practices for biorepository activities. The guidelines are meant to be a living document that is modified as new technologies, procedures, and regulations evolve.

The establishment of best-practice guidelines represents a tremendous advance toward optimizing the utility of biospecimens for wider ranging research applications while protecting patient privacy and safety. However, the added responsibilities for the biobanks mean increasing difficulties for small, investigator-driven efforts in terms of cost, infrastructure, and personnel. More institutions are moving toward centralized repositories, which can serve the needs of multiple research groups more efficiently and cost effectively. Because tissue diagnostics and laboratory analysis of body fluids lies within the realm of pathology, pathologists are increasingly and appropriately being called upon to administer centralized repositories. Centralization of archival efforts requires careful consideration of the needs and requirements of the research community. Other factors that require careful consideration are the quantity, types, and future suitability of patients' specimens (and derivatives thereof) that are to be archived; the delineation of space and equipment; the establishment of informatics support; and the logistics of dissemination of specimens and data for research projects.

Figure 4-1 depicts the basic pathway of biospecimen procurement, processing, annotation, and distribution for translational research. Table 4-1 lists the basic aspects of biorepository operations that must be considered when developing an institutional biorepository that encompasses all aspects of the flowchart in Figure 4-1. The degree to which these aspects can be optimized is determined by the amount of dedicated effort put forth; the quality of communication among biobanking personnel, clinicians, and researchers; the quality and quantity of informatics support; and the strength of institutional support.

Determining the Scope of the Biorepository: What Specimens Will Be Archived?

For a biorepository to function well as a valuable research resource, its development from beginning to

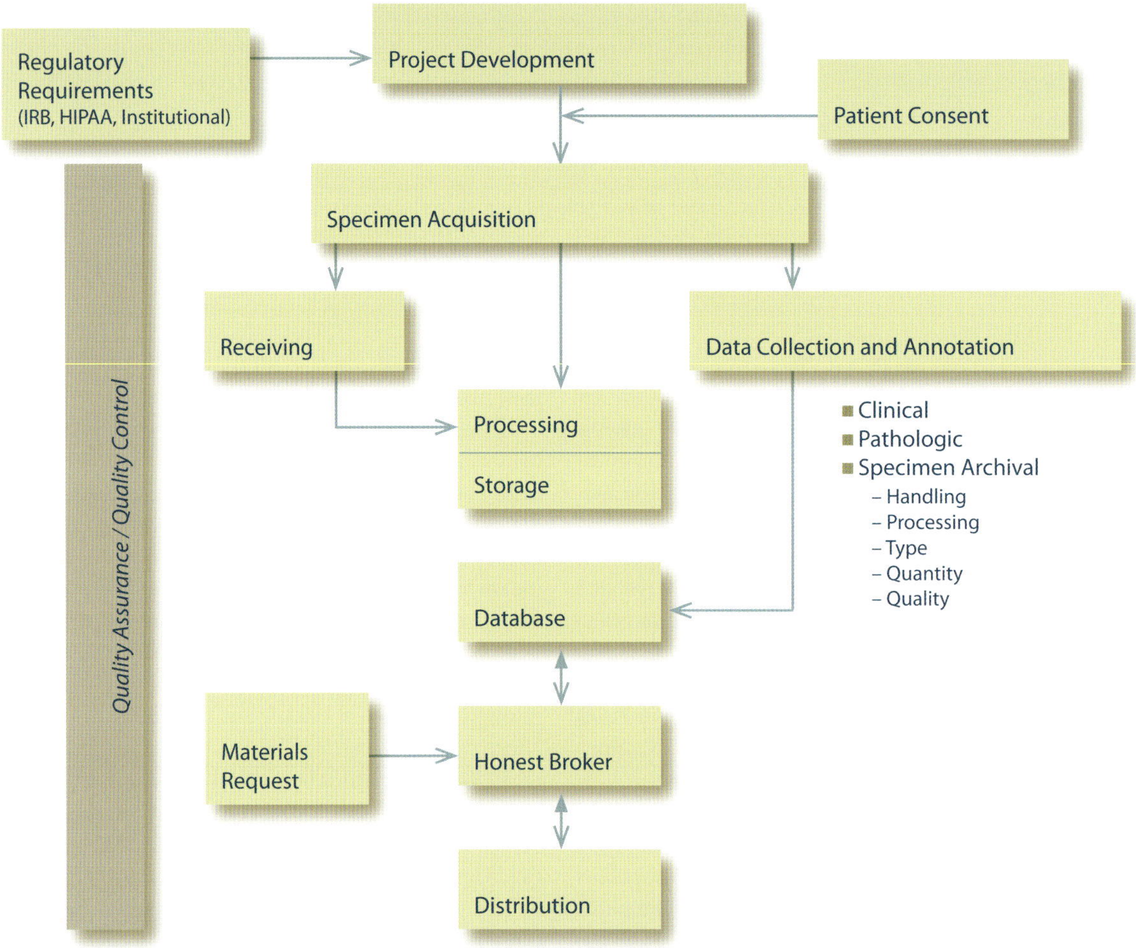

Figure 4-1. Flowchart of specimen acquisition, processing, annotation, and distribution.
Abbreviations: IRB, Institutional Review Board; HIPAA, Health Insurance Portability and Accountability Act of 1996.

end must be intentional. Its purpose and scope, along with the types of specimens to be collected, should be defined in order to establish infrastructure needs. For example, a biorepository that is limited to obtaining remnant surgical tissue from one type of disease may be able to operate efficiently within the space of an existing pathology suite. In contrast, a repository that collects from clinic patients a range of body fluids (eg, blood, urine, cerebrospinal fluid) that are suitable for proteomic studies, in addition to fresh tissue from surgeries, will require much larger storage capacity, more specialized handling and cryopreservation techniques, and a dedicated team of personnel.

Because the specimen-handling methods for most applications use common best practices,[2] centralization of archiving efforts is optimal. Centralization has the advantages of (1) improved cost efficiency through reduced redundancy, (2) unified and standardized protocols that allow for meaningful comparison of results of separate studies, (3) dedicated personnel specifically trained for collection and handling of specimens, (4) conservation of space, and (5) improved clinical annotation of specimens and linkage of data. However, the advantages must be balanced with practicality, recognizing that a facility that attempts to "do everything" is not very practical. Therefore, identifying and communicating with the researchers who will be served by the repository is essential during the planning stages.

Almost any specimen removed from or produced by a human or animal can be preserved and archived in a manner conducive to research. Anything from hair and toenails (dry storage) to buccal swabs and body fluids to tissue samples removed by biopsy or surgery have been subject to collection for research purposes. The most commonly archived specimens are those samples that have the broadest range of utility for research; these include blood and its derivatives, urine, and fresh or fixed tissue samples. Table 4-2 has a more extensive list of specimen types and possible derivatives suitable for biorepository storage and research.

Table 4-1. General Considerations When Designing and Developing a Biorepository

Topic	Items to Consider
Size and location	Storage/laboratory/office/information technology/ special processing and analysis
Personnel requirement	Director, management, staff, clinical coordinators
Procurement sources	Clinic, operating room, home collection
Patient enrollment	Regulatory compliance, IRB, HIPAA, patient care and safety
Communication	Clinic, researcher
Storage equipment	-80°C freezer, liquid nitrogen, slides, paraffin blocks
Equipment for processing and analysis	Centrifuges, safety cabinets
Safety procedures	Rules and regulations, fire, hazardous, infectious
Training	Safety regulations, procedures
Shipping/receiving	Shipping regulations
Quality assurance/quality control	—
Collected specimens types	Liquids, tissue, organ site, normal controls
Clinical, pathological, and specimen archival data	—
Informatics/information technology	Data storage, data exchange
Institutional support	Long-term sustainability
Financial support	Charge back, fee for service
Backup storage	—
Monitoring and alarm systems	Staff to respond after hours
Future research	—
Standard operating procedures	—

Abbreviations: IRB, Institutional Review Board; HIPAA, Health Insurance Portability and Accountability Act of 1996.

For any procurement effort that involves biological samples removed from humans, the involvement of a pathologist is essential, especially for tissues removed surgically for diagnostic or therapeutic purposes. The primary responsibility of the pathologist is diagnosis; in the case of cancer resections, this includes proper grading and staging of disease. Any tissue in excess of that required to fulfill this responsibility can be targeted for archiving, provided proper patient consent and Institutional Review Board (IRB) approval have been obtained (see chapter 8, *Biorepository Informed Consent Process,* and chapter 5, *Flow of Biospecimens,* "Participant Identification and Informed Consent"). The pathologist is best qualified to determine which tissues are most representative of the disease and appropriate benign tissue that can be removed without compromising patient care, and is in the best position to obtain the material in a rapid, nonbiased manner. It is also advantageous to have a pathologist or pathology personnel involved with archiving of body fluids. The advantages include centralization of processing and storage, improved linkage with pathology diagnoses and laboratory results, and separation of research interests from the interests of patient care.

Careful consideration of the types and numbers of specimens to be archived within the institutional biorepository is important in the planning phase in order to better determine (1) the amount of space required for physical storage, (2) the space required for receiving and processing, (3) the design and location of the space requirements relative to the site(s) of procurement (ie, surgical suite versus clinic), (4) the equipment required for processing and storage of specimens, and (5) the personnel required (addressed in chapter 2, *Getting Started: Developing an Institutional Resource Within the Pathology Department*).

Determining Biobank Space and System Requirements

Biospecimens must be stored in a manner that stabilizes them and prevents degradation and desiccation. For body fluid specimens, this generally means storage in a cryopreservation unit (-80°C or colder). Depending on research interests, all components of blood specimens (serum and/or plasma, buffy coat,

Table 4-2. Processing and Storage Conditions for Various Commonly Collected Biospecimen Types

Tissue	Source	Fractionation	Storage	Derivatives
Blood	Clinic, surgery	Whole blood	-80°C	DNA, RNA
		Serum	-80°C	Protein, metabolites, DNA
		Plasma	-80°C	Protein, metabolites, DNA
		Buffy coat / WBCs	-80°C, LN_2	DNA, cell line
		Blood clot	-80°C	DNA
Bone marrow	Surgery, autopsy	—	-80°C	Protein, metabolites, DNA, RNA
Cerebrospinal fluid	Clinic, surgery	Whole	-80°C	Protein, DNA, RNA
		Supernatant	-80°C	Protein, metabolites, DNA, RNA
		Cells	-80°C, LN_2	Protein, metabolites, DNA, RNA
Fine-needle aspirate	Clinic, surgery	—	-80°C	Protein, metabolites, DNA, RNA
Hair	Off-site, clinic, surgery	—	-80°C	Protein, metabolites, minerals
Saliva	Off-site, clinic, surgery	—	RT, -80°C	Protein, metabolites, DNA, RNA
Skin	Surgery, autopsy	—	-80°C	Protein, DNA, RNA, cell line
Solid tissue	Surgery, autopsy	Fresh	RT, 4°C	Xenograft, primary culture, cell line
		Frozen	LN_2	Tissue sections, protein, metabolites, DNA, RNA
		RNAse later	RT, -80°C	RNA
	Surgery, autopsy, pathology archive	FFPE	RT	Tissue sections, protein, DNA, RNA
Sputum / buccal	Off-site, clinic, surgery	—	RT, -80°C	Protein, metabolites, DNA, RNA
Toenails	Off-site, clinic, surgery	—	-80°C	Protein, metabolites, minerals
Urine	Off-site, clinic, surgery	Whole urine	-80°C	Protein, metabolites, DNA, RNA, microbes
		Supernatant	-80°C	Protein, metabolites, DNA, RNA
		Sediment	-80°C	DNA, RNA, microbes

Abbreviations: WBCs, white blood cells; LN_2, liquid nitrogen; RT, room temperature; FFPE, formalin-fixed paraffin-embedded.

red blood cells) should be separated and stored. On average, a 10-mL sample of blood collected in a red-top Vacutainer tube can produce 4 to 5 mL of serum. Thus, multiple, separate, serum aliquot tubes may result from a single collection. In addition, the blood clot from a serum tube can be used to isolate chromosomal DNA, resulting in the generation of additional derivative samples of DNA. Aliquoting of samples up front is optimal for avoiding unnecessary freeze–thaw cycles of the sample residuals when removing small amounts for research distribution or analysis. The typical upright cryopreservation unit requires 24 square feet of space in order to house and safely access the samples; it can store up to 32,000 tubes (0.5–1.5 mL) arranged in storage boxes and rack units. Depending on expected usage, freezer space could fill up relatively quickly. In order to maximally conserve space within the freezers, it is necessary to have a system that tracks open storage slots for potential refill as tubes are removed from the archive. Even so, accrual of specimens usually exceeds usage, at least in the beginning of repository efforts. Therefore, the freezer facility needs ample space for expansion.

To illustrate, the Prostate Cancer Awareness Week blood biorepository at the University of Colorado Anschutz Medical Campus (UCAMC) collects blood samples from participants being screened for prostate cancer across several sites in the United States (www.prostateconditions.org). More than 10,000 tubes of serum are collected every year. The approximately 150,000 total samples that have been obtained from 15 years of the program require 6 freezers to house and occupy 144 square feet of biorepository space.

Urine specimens also often are separated into sediment and supernatant fractions and stored as aliquots. Cerebrospinal fluid or other fluids may result in fewer aliquots and therefore a smaller footprint per subject. Cell samples (aspirates) or tissues collected fresh should optimally be stored below the glass point of water (-130°C) to avoid desiccation over time. This requires either ultra-low freezer units or storage in liquid nitrogen. For the latter, space reserved for portable liquid nitrogen canisters is necessary unless a centralized tank with pigtail connections to multiple units is available.

Safely and securely archiving and managing a large collection of biospecimens requires careful consideration in designing the space. Frozen specimens, paraffin-embedded specimens, and glass slides should be separately aggregated. Archival space requires fire protection systems and proper control of temperature and humidity. Maintaining temperature conditions to exchange the heat generated from a large collection of freezers may require modification of the normal building environmental controls. For example, the freezer bank at UCAMC houses 100 freezers in a single large room. To maintain reasonable temperature and air flow in the facility, additional cooling units were installed that replace the air every few minutes. Furthermore, to guarantee specimen preservation during a power outage, dedicated backup generators or other alternate power supplies with sufficient capacity are essential. Round-the-clock monitoring requires, at a minimum, that an electronic monitoring system is in place that automatically dials out to report temperature failures of individual units. For example, the UCAMC biorepository has a temperature-monitoring system that can record the temperature of each freezer unit and the overall space in real time and can be accessed through a web-based interface. Biorepository staff are trained to deal with emergencies and are on call on rotating schedules to have 24/7 coverage to respond to alarms. A daily manual walk-through to check space and freezer conditions supplements electronic monitoring. For security and HIPAA considerations, access to the repository storage space and records should be limited to authorized personnel via keycard or other controlled-access mechanism.

Tissues that have been formalin-fixed and paraffin-embedded (FFPE) can be maintained at room temperature provided that the temperature does not exceed 25°C (77°F) and the blocks are protected from dust and excessive humidity.[3] Tissue block and slide storage can often be accomplished efficiently in smaller areas; however, tissue blocks usually require additional processing, such as histologic sectioning, creation of tissue arrays, or laser capture microdissection before distribution (see "Ancillary Core Laboratory Services" below). Thus, if these services are not provided by an ancillary or partnering laboratory, additional space for these associated activities may be necessary.

Receiving and Processing

The physical storage units for archiving biospecimens represent only a part of the space requirements for a well-functioning biorepository. Adequate space is also required for personnel to receive and process specimens before archiving or distribution. This includes a clean area with computer access for specimen receipt and entry into the database and a benchtop area with centrifuge, equipment, and supplies for creating archival units (eg, tubes, blocks, cell pellets). In addition, this space can also serve to prepare specimens for packaging and distribution to investigators. The space requirements will vary according to the magnitude of the repository and the number of staff it must accommodate.

Location and Design Considerations

Location and design of the repository are important considerations. Ideally, the repository, or at least the receiving and processing area, should be physically located as close as possible to the source of the biospecimens. For body fluids and fresh tissues, the sooner the specimen can be placed in cryopreservation after removal from the body, the better. For collection of fresh tissues from surgical resection specimens, this usually requires interception of the specimen in a pathology grossing or frozen-section room and collaboration with the pathologist to obtain suitable lesional and paired normal tissue as rapidly as possible without compromising the patient's care. In this situation, the delineation of separate areas for tissue procurement, while ideal, may not be practical. Use of a portable tray or cart loaded with tissue cassettes, cryomolds, embedding media, dissection instruments, tubes, and a container of liquid nitrogen or other freezing medium for quick freezing may be all that is practical to obtain and transfer the specimens to the storage facility. Preferably, the storage facility itself is also as close as possible to the specimen handling facility. Determining the best location for centralization of blood and body fluid processing is more problematic.

Delays in processing and freezing can compromise the validity of results for some applications.[4] One must balance timeliness of processing with practicality and feasibility. For example, although processing at the site of procurement may be ideal, this is not always feasible when procurement is performed at external institutions where technical expertise and/or required equipment and facilities are not readily available. In addition, procurement and processing on site by local staff at multiple institutions might introduce a greater degree of specimen variability. For some research studies, timely (overnight) transport to a centralized processing area for body fluids may be desired. Regardless of whether specimens are immediately processed on site or at a centralized laboratory, the goal in collection always should be that specimens are collected according to a standardized protocol. However, sometimes exceptions to and deviations from the standard protocol are inevitable. Therefore, to ensure high quality of research specimens, proper and detailed annotation is necessary to record critical information such as collection, processing, and storage times. Although the biorepository should be the driving force behind standardization, involvement of clinical personnel will be critical to ensure proper handling, transfer, and annotation of specimens. An up-to-date copy of the repository's manual of standard operating procedures (SOPs) should be present at all locations that collect or process biospecimens. The SOP manual should describe in detail the procedures for:

- Obtaining informed consent from patients
- Obtaining proper IRB approvals
- Collecting and handling of biospecimens by type
- Clinical and pathologic annotation of biospecimens
- Quality assurance measures
- Coordination of requests for biospecimens and associated data
- Distribution of biomaterials and data
- Safety and regulatory guidelines
- Emergency procedures and information

Ancillary Core Laboratory Services

The ultimate goal of a comprehensive biorepository is to provide the highest quality, nonbiased biospecimens that are uniformly processed and prepared to meet the needs of research teams having wide-ranging interests and specimen requirements. Biospecimens may be subjected to a multitude of analytical applications, including pathobiology, genetics, gene expression, proteomics, metabolomics, and pharmacokinetics. As much as possible, centralization of specimen processing and preparation by the biorepository facility is warranted. Centralized sample processing ensures uniformity across multiple studies, thereby allowing for better reproducibility and comparability of analytical results. It also protects the archive from fragmentation, loss, and waste from unneeded transfer of specimens from laboratory to laboratory, thus stretching the resource. A properly organized biorepository will need to provide the following additional services beyond specimen collection and distribution: (1) aliquoting and fractionation of liquid samples, (2) lesional dissection or histologic preparation of tissue samples, (3) creation of tissue microarrays (TMAs), (4) isolation of DNA or RNA, and (5) imaging of tissues. For some services, integration into the biorepository operation is optimal, whereas other services are best provided through close collaborations with other core facilities. Ideally, these interactions and collaborations should be set up before collection and processing protocols are developed so as to enable input regarding special requirements for collection and/or processing of specimens that highly specialized services such as proteomics, metabolomics, and genomics might require.

Histology and Immunohistochemistry

In our experience, a close relationship with a full-service histology laboratory is crucial for the effective provision of high-quality tissue samples either collected fresh and then frozen or obtained from archival remnant pathologic tissue. In some cases, the biorepository itself may provide basic histology services. In other instances, the facility interacts with or is part of an institution's pathology department or laboratory that is certified according to the Clinical Laboratory Improvement Amendments (CLIA) and meets the requirements of the College of American Pathologists. The biorepository at UCAMC is physically located adjacent to the Research Histology Laboratory within the Department of Pathology. The laboratory is approximately 800 square feet and performs routine histology—including microtomy, cryomicrotomy of frozen tissues, and routine and special staining—for biospecimens that are to be used for research. A pathologist works closely with the laboratory personnel to review specimens for adequacy, lesional integrity, tissue macrodissection or microdissection if necessary, and to identify regions of interest in tissues for subsequent processing into TMAs. The laboratory also provides immunohistochemistry services if requested by investigators, including antibody optimization and staining using a number of different platforms.

Tissue Imaging and Laser Capture Microdissection

Research projects often involve isolation of specific cell types and/or specific lesions from tissue specimens as a starting material for DNA or RNA isolation. Macrocapture or laser capture microdissection techniques needed for this process require specialized protocols, equipment, and personnel and are best overseen by a pathologist. Biorepositories are well suited to provide these services, either as part of their operation or as ancillary core services. There has been an increased need to document high-quality digital reproductions of stained tissue sections for future reference or to provide a platform for individually annotating histologic sections for particular research purposes. Improvements in computer-assisted digital imaging have made it into a powerful tool for pathologic review between pathologists, for annotation of pathologic features, and for digital image analysis techniques. Ideally, an imaging system that allows for imaging of entire tissue sections at high resolution that can be displayed over a web-based viewer and annotated for precise areas to be dissected is used for documentation of individual tissue sections. Several imaging systems are commercially available (eg, Aperio, Vista, CA; Ventana Medical Systems, Tucson, AZ; Hamamatsu, Hamamatsu City, Japan; Zeiss, Gottingen, Germany; DMetrix, Tucson, AZ) that provide images that can be annotated for pathology or to designate specific areas within tissue blocks for subsequent transfer to a TMA (see below). Laser capture microdissection systems (eg, Applied Biosystems, Carlsbad, CA; Zeiss, Gottingen, Germany) are also available to allow dissection of individual cells from paraffin-embedded or frozen tissue sections for subsequent extraction of DNA or RNA. Proper information technology infrastructure, with sufficient server and storage capacity, and qualified personnel trained in information technology and imaging technology are essential to provide these services.

Tissue Microarrays

Tissue samples obtained from biopsies or surgical resections represent a precious but finite resource for understanding the pathobiology of disease, evaluating the expression of biomarkers by either immunohistochemistry or in situ hybridization, or quantifying the severity of disease and/or disease characteristics in target tissues. Although a number of sections can be taken for analysis from a single tissue sample, eventually the tissue sample will be exhausted. Furthermore, studies that require staining or analysis of large numbers of tissue samples can be labor intensive, expensive in terms of cost and time, and inefficient. These problems can be minimized by the generation of tissue arrays to help preserve tissue and allow for rapid screening of multiple samples in the same analysis. To streamline and expedite immunohistochemical studies when numerous samples are to be analyzed, the creation of tissue microarrays can be a cost-effective alternative. This requires harvesting tissue from numerous paraffin blocks using a coring needle and then transferring the cores to a new block in which the cores are arrayed in rows and then sectioned onto a single slide. Participation of a pathologist is crucial in order to identify the precise areas to be cored and transferred from the original tissue sample and to continually evaluate the integrity of the sections from the TMAs as they are used. Manual and automated apparatuses are available commercially (Beecher Instruments, Sun Prairie, WI; Veridiam, Oceanside, CA).

Equipment and Special Handling

The range of equipment needed to successfully manage and maintain a successful biorepository operation depends on the type of specimens that are collected and the scope of processing services to be made available. Procurement of biofluids such as blood and urine usually does not require processing equipment beyond what is available in the standard clinic, such as a benchtop centrifuge that can handle centrifugation of 10-mL to 50-mL tubes at relatively low speeds, pipettes for sample aliquoting, and transport containers with ice. However, as discussed previously, collection of tissue specimens from surgical procedures requires a pathologist's participation and access to the point-of-specimen-delivery within the pathology department. At a minimum, a portable tray or cart can be loaded with tissue cassettes, cryomolds, embedding media, dissection instruments, tubes, and an appropriate container for quick freezing and transport to the cryopreservation unit. Transport containers suited and approved for liquid nitrogen or dry ice are needed for secure and safe transport of frozen specimens from clinic or pathology suite to the laboratory or long-term storage. Transport vessels for liquid nitrogen (Dewars are available from general laboratory supply companies) are preferable for transporting frozen solid-tissue specimens. If liquid nitrogen is not available, Styrofoam containers that can hold pelleted dry ice can be used as an alternative. For fluid specimens, dry ice transportation is sufficient in most cases. Suitable secondary containers for spill containment are required for transporting specimens in fixative (eg, formalin). For biobanking operations with sufficient resources, robotic systems for all aspects of specimen archiving and retrieval and biofluid aliquoting are available (eg, Hamilton Storage Technologies, Hopkinton, MA; Qiagen, Valencia, CA; Eppendorf, Hauppauge, NY).

Table 4-2 lists the optimal storage temperature for different specimen types and derivatives. For best preservation, snap-frozen tissue should be stored in liquid nitrogen either in a full-liquid format (tissue is stored in the liquid phase at -190°C) or in vapor format (tissue is stored in the vapor phase at -130°C). Each has advantages and disadvantages. Liquid storage has better capabilities for maintaining constant temperature throughout the container than does vapor phase storage. The standard, however, is shifting to vapor storage because newer generation vapor phase storage options have improved significantly and are now capable of better maintenance of constant temperature throughout the container. For safety reasons, vapor is preferred by some, because tubes stored in the liquid phase of liquid nitrogen sometimes fill with liquid nitrogen that expands upon removal from liquid phase, resulting in tubes that rupture or explode. In some cases, mechanical ultralow freezers (-130°C) are a reliable and cost-effective alternative. Compared with mechanical storage, liquid nitrogen is more costly but is also less sensitive to power interruption because it can maintain its temperature for longer periods of time.

Although many research requirements can be fulfilled by simply supplying aliquots of a biofluid specimen or a portion of a frozen or FFPE tissue specimen, derivative sample types often have to be isolated (such as DNA or RNA) from a specimen source, or a particular archival tissue specimen requires special processing (eg, enrichment for tumor cells through microdissection, provide unstained sections for immunohistochemistry, etc). To fulfill this need, a comprehensive biorepository may choose to offer these services or associate with other core facilities that provide these services. For a biorepository that archives and provides tissue specimens for research, access to basic histology services is essential to conserve the tissue and provide uniform processing quality. If this cannot be accomplished through collaboration with a dedicated histology laboratory, then the biorepository should be equipped with basic microtomes for sectioning of FFPE tissue blocks; flotation baths; mounting, staining, and coverslipping stations; and a cryotome for sectioning frozen tissues. Sources for histology equipment include Fisher Scientific (Pittsburgh, PA), Life Science Products (Frederick, CO), StatLab (McKinney, TX), and Mopec (Oak Park, MI). To provide even basic histology services of good quality requires the expertise of personnel who are appropriately trained.

Depending on the quantity of specimens, automation for nucleic acid isolation should be considered as a cost-effective alternative for manual processing. Automation (such as the Qiacube, Qiagen, Valencia, CA) also allows for better standardization and quicker throughput times because instruments can run after normal workday hours. Quantity and quality of isolates should be confirmed before distribution: analysis using a Nanodrop spectrophotometer (Thermal Scientific, Wilmington, DE) allows for quick assessment of quantity and purity of nucleic acid and protein isolates using small amounts of material. Additional analyses for quality assurance and quality control (QA/QC) are often required: a microfluidics-based platform approach (such as the Agilent Bioanalyzer, Agilent Technologies, Santa Clara, CA) or polymerase chain reaction (PCR) platforms (such as Applied Biosystems Taqman or Roche Lightcycler) provide excellent results in a timely fashion. If PCR methods are used for analysis or QA/QC, proper space separation is needed to prevent contamination problems. Our biorepository uses -80°C storage for tissue derivatives such as DNA and RNA. Storage at higher temperature (-30°C) has been used successfully by others. Technologies for dry storage of DNA specimens have been developed and validated and are commercially available (Biomatrica, Inc, San Diego, CA; Qiagen, Valencia, CA; IntegenX, Pleasanton, CA).

Although there are economic considerations that favor dry storage for a biorepository with active research distribution, it is not always the most practical storage. Some studies opt for creating immortalized lymphocytes to guarantee future availability of chromosomal DNA. For such activities, in vitro cell cultures from tissue specimens need to be prepared and maintained in a separate laboratory space equipped with a biosafety cabinet and CO_2 incubators. Created cell lines should be stored in liquid nitrogen.

Conclusion

Establishment of a comprehensive biorepository facility in support of translational research requires careful planning, attention to detail, and considerable institutional support. Biobanking operations are expensive, require dedicated and well-trained personnel, and have specialized infrastructural requirements. As awareness of the strengths and limitations of the use of biospecimens in research grows, so does the recognition that adherence to proper best-practices procedures and regulations is crucial for the success of any biorepository.

References

1. 132nd National Cancer Advisory Board. XX Summary of Meeting; November 30–December 1, 2004; Department of Health and Human Services, Public Health Service, National Cancer Institute, Bethesda, MD.
2. Office of Biorepositories and Biospecimen Research, National Cancer Institute. *NCI Best Practices for Biospecimen Resources.* Washington, DC: National Institutes of Health, US Department of Health and Human Services; 2011. http://biospecimens.cancer.gov/practices/2011bp.asp. Accessed March 31, 2014.
3. Xie R, Chung J-Y, Ylaya K, et al. Factors influencing the degradation of archival formalin-fixed paraffin-embedded tissue sections. *J Histochem Cytochem.* 2011;59:356-365.
4. Elliott P, Peakman TC. The UK Biobank sample handling and storage protocol for the collection, processing and archiving of human blood and urine. *Int J Epidemiol.* 2008;37:234-244.

Chapter 5

Flow of Biospecimens: From the Clinic or Operating Room To and From the Biospecimen Repository

Daniel Rohrer
David W. Chesla
Scott D. Jewell

Introduction

The procedures for collection, processing, storage, and distribution of biospecimens vary considerably from institution to institution and often within institutions. These procedures are dependent on the degree of organization, support, management, and the specific biospecimen repository (biorepository) model. The biospecimen collection process for a central biorepository can involve several departments such as the clinic, clinical and anatomic pathology, and the operating room (OR). A central campus-wide biorepository developed for use by many investigators faces both similar and different responsibilities from a single use (investigator managed) biorepository. The goals of a centralized biorepository include efficiency in the proper management of biospecimen collection, processing, storage, and distribution; adherence to best practices; assurance in human subjects regulations; and increase in the sharing of biospecimens and their associated data with the institution or investigators, rather than a silo approach to the management of biospecimens. This chapter will focus primarily on the institution centralized biorepository model and the processes of collecting the biospecimens.

A centralized biorepository model must have the support of the leadership of the institution. The central biorepository purpose and goals should determine it to be a valuable asset to the institution in lieu of the provisions for facilities and financial support. The first choice for managing a central biorepository is often the pathology department and secondly an office of medical research. The breadth and sophistication of the central biorepository is defined by its purpose and goals, which can vary considerably. The range of activities can include screening and consenting prospective patients, and collection, processing, storage, and distribution of the biospecimens; or a biorepository can include only the biobanking functions (ie, receipt, storage, and distribution). Because of the increased focus on quality research results for basic and translational research, academic institutions are recognizing that a well-defined and well-managed central biorepository is an important institutional research resource.

Structure and Functions of the Biorepository

Centralized biorepositories are often directly involved in the collection of biospecimens through dedicated procurement personnel in the clinical environments who manage the daily monitoring and communication with key clinical personnel. Close proximity of the biorepository and its personnel to the collection areas is beneficial for acquiring, processing, and storing biospecimens in a timely and efficient manner. Biorepositories that are separate from the site of specimen collection should include the use of wet ice and expedited courier services to transport tissues in a timely manner to maintain the quality of the tissue. Proper collection procedures include participants' protocols, informed consent (Institutional Review Board [IRB], federal regulations), tissue evaluation, dissection, and timely processing procedures. When a biorepository is separate from the collection site, proper temperature control during transportation is required. The model of collection and management of human biospecimens should include the local, state, and federal regulations as they apply to the biorepository's structure and function. This is more seamlessly accomplished through the centralized biorepository model. The term *biorepository* can therefore expand to *biospecimen resources* because this centralized model provides a more comprehensive approach to managing biospecimens. A central biorepository must put into place both emergency and disaster plans for the biorepository, an aspect often overlooked by individual investigators. To summarize, the biospecimen resource or biorepository would include the informed consent, collection, processing, banking, distribution, and final disposition of biospecimens.

Standardization of Biospecimen Collection Using Biospecimen Kits

A widespread concern in the collection of biospecimens is the degree of variation in the collection procedures. Standardization of biospecimen collection kits is an effective way to ensure greater consistency in biospecimen collection. These kits often contain all the materials necessary to properly collect, preserve, and ship biospecimens to the biorepository. Collection kits will vary depending on the type of specimens, temperature conditions, and shipping methods. Collection kits can be used for institutional collection procedures as well because they contain the proper materials, but they are essential if the biospecimens are coming from source sites outside the institution.

The construction of kits must satisfy all applicable laws and regulations, such as the International Air Transport Association (IATA)[1] and/or Department of Transportation[2] regulations. Persons affiliated with the biorepository can consult these agencies for information concerning transportation regulations and the classifications of packages and specimens for shipment. In general, kits are composed of an outer corrugated shell, an inner insulated container, primary collection receptacles, packing material, and temperature-regulating materials such as dry ice or freezer packs (Figure 5-1). Kits do not generally contain surgical tools or routine receptacles used in standard-of-care surgical procedures.

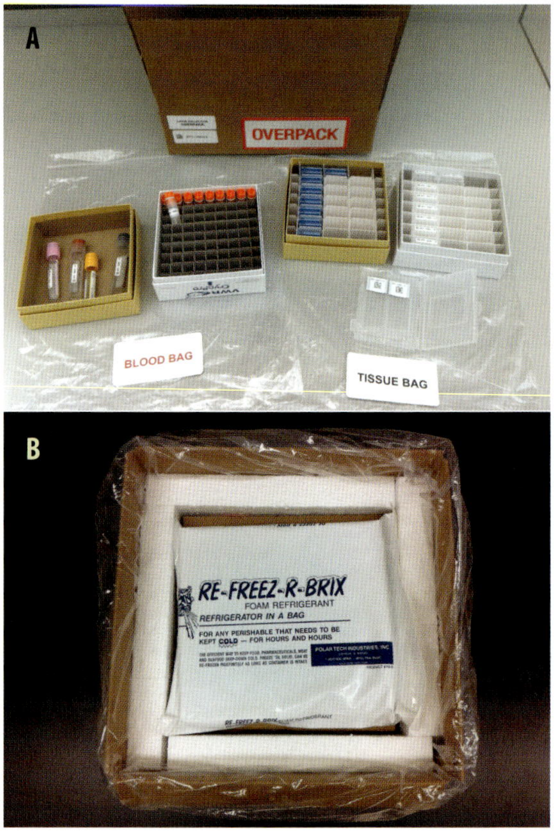

Figure 5-1. Examples of kit contents (A) and packaging for shipment (B).

Examples of biospecimen collection kit items include procurement materials, tissue cassettes, vials, tubes, cryotubes, reagents, container labels, shipping labels, and data forms. In blood collections, blood tubes can be considered for phlebotomy if the process of getting these to the phlebotomist is not in itself too complicated. Often, blood collections can rely on the blood tube supply of the phlebotomist, and a form of reimbursement can be established if needed. The standardization of biospecimen collections within an institution can be controlled better if kits are developed; however, depending on the structure of the operations, institutions may also use the existing clinical material sources (eg, phlebotomy tubes) as well as bulk supplies available to the procurement personnel.

Careful planning is necessary when determining the scheme for biospecimen labels and the subsequent downstream use. This scheme should, at a minimum, allow for a unique identifier for each "parent biospecimen" and for each "child aliquot" or derivative throughout the entire bank. Identifiers must never repeat. Care should be taken to plan for the future in allowing the scheme to grow with the bank (ie, not limiting the identifier through character length or other restrictions). The identifier should be anonymous, in that identifying information (either to the patient or the source site) should not be embedded directly in the code. Presently, bar-coded unique identifiers on labels is the standard in tracking the path of the biospecimen from collection to processing to storage to distribution. The ability to assign new biospecimen numbers to derivatives of primary specimens that do not link to the parent sample through the identifier code (rather, in the inventory system only) is of increasing value for downstream distribution to investigators. The biorepository inventory information system should contain flexible biospecimen numbering assignment capability while ensuring connectivity back to the primary biospecimen.

For institutions where tissues are transported from the OR to the pathology department, cooled containers or wet-ice buckets should be used to maintain lower temperatures to minimize cold ischemia preanalytic variables. To date, published data have not definitively determined a best practice for biospecimen analytes, but the general consensus is that controlled conditions are best. Distance and weather conditions can affect sample quality during transportation if not properly controlled. Because tissues coming from surgical procedures are still part of the clinical process, the management of the tissue specimen for research should involve the clinical and pathology departments in order to determine if deviations from the clinical practice are allowable. The same considerations may need to be given for blood collections as well, because practices in proteomics may require rapid processing to minimize degradation of proteins by proteases. After the point of collection, it is critical to hand off biospecimens to the biorepository/procurement technologist for quick processing to protect against degradation. Electronic temperature data loggers are tools that can be helpful both to assess and track the temperature conditions that biospecimens encounter, in addition to determining whether the biospecimen shipping containers are functioning as planned.

The use of collection kits must be managed, at a minimum, through the tracking of courier shipments and expiration dates of materials in the kits. This is most efficiently and effectively handled in a tracking database using unique kit identifiers, with unique identifiers for prelabeled contents linked to each kit identifier, with expiration dates and lot numbers of contents, date of shipment, associated courier tracking number, and the destination. Kits (and their contents) should be linked to a specific participant collection event. This linkage to a collection event is generally completed by the procurement technician. A tracking database allows the biorepository personnel to track the usage of the kits by source sites or internal use and maintain adequate inventory of collection supplies.

Participant Identification and Informed Consent

The person (eg, clinical research coordinator, nurse, or physician) implementing the consent process for patients must be trained in human subjects research and specifically in biospecimen collection for the biorepository. The informed consent will cover all of the general statements to provide the patient with a clear and thorough understanding of what they are being asked to donate. Patients should be given ample opportunity to consider donation, and participants should have the opportunity to withdraw the donation of their biospecimens and annotated clinical data at any time. Consenting for the collection of biospecimens poses minimal risk in almost every situation of routine scheduled phlebotomy or from surgical standard-of-care procedures. If a surgical procedure is being planned to specifically obtain biospecimens for research purposes, a full IRB review and medical assessment of risk should be required. The consent form should have specific features that help the participant to understand the measure of protection of their identity and may also include discussion on information such as the Genetic Information Nondiscrimination Act of 2008 and a Certificate of Confidentiality from the National Institutes of Health (NIH).[3,4] Critical to the collection of biospecimens, after consent, is the communication that the consent has been given and approved by the participant. Some IRBs and ethical groups prefer to have the consent in place before an attempt to collect a biospecimen. Under other IRB informed-consent approvals, either a presurgical or a postsurgical consent process is acceptable.[5] To ensure proper chain of custody, a document system (preferably electronic) is advisable to track each process from consent to distribution.

The optimal time and situation for obtaining the informed consent for the biorepository can depend on the amount of information the health care team and the patient have regarding diagnosis and prognosis. Practical considerations also affect the consenting process, in particular the availability of staff trained to oversee the informed consent process. The most flexible and comprehensive approach involves providing an informative letter and a copy of the biorepository consent at the time the patient meets with a surgeon or clinical staff member to plan a procedure or health care plan. Biorepository/research staff can then follow up with the patient before the procedure/surgical date in the clinic or by telephone, or on the morning of surgery within the presurgical waiting/holding area, in order to answer any questions and obtain the final signed consent. The research staff should have copies of the documents available for the patient in the event the patient does not bring them. In some circumstances where the surgeon is involved in the consenting process or research personnel are available at the time of a procedure or treatment planning, consent may be obtained at a clinic or during an office visit.

Obtaining the consent in advance helps to remove any urgency and avoids patient anxiety in acquiring consent immediately before the clinical procedure. Tracking the status of the consent from the patient through the biospecimen collection and processing assists in avoiding duplication of efforts, on one hand, and omission of patients from consenting, on the other hand. Individual institutional guidelines through the IRB may prohibit biospecimen collections outside of 30 days of informed consent. In such situations, patients may need to re-consent, and the workflow may need to be altered to accommodate an extended duration between office/clinic visit and the date of surgery. These durations are most often encountered in institutions that offer solid-organ transplant services.

Few health care systems have one electronic medical record that covers all out-patient (physicians'/surgeons' offices) and in-patient (hospital/surgical center) encounters for the entire system. If electronic tracking of consent is not available or practical, maintaining a "consent log" by the research staff may be adequate. The consent logs should track those patients who have consented, declined, or were approached and given information but have not yet responded. It is good practice to transmit this information to the procurement teams, surgical pathology department, and OR teams on the day of the procedure to ensure consented biospecimens are collected and declined consents are honored. Transmittal of information regarding the patient's willingness to participate and donate biospecimens can be accomplished by direct verbal communication, patient chart labels placed by staff, or placement of transport materials, such as an appropriately labeled insulated receptacle, in the procedure or OR suite. Finally, the patient's consent may be gathered postoperatively in the hospital or possibly at a postoperative follow-up appointment, which often happens when the diagnosis and treatment plan is better defined.[5] If a delay in consenting occurs, the "remnant" biospecimens should be held and not distributed for research until the informed consent is obtained. A plan should be in place to destroy biospecimens when the patient's consent has not been acquired.

When informed consent is to be obtained on the day of surgery, one effective method to identify the potential eligibility of surgical cases is to evaluate the OR schedule several days in advance. Then verify the procedure is scheduled to take place on the afternoon before the day of surgery, or in same-day cases check the early morning schedules. Eligibility for collection and biobanking should meet three criteria:

- Is the tissue valuable to research (a specific project or general use)?
- Can the patient be consented to participate in the donation of the biospecimen?
- Will the surgical procedure likely yield sufficient tissue for research?

The postsurgical model of informed consent is based on two factors. The first is that if the tissue is being removed as part of a clinical procedure, it can be held until consent is obtained within a reasonable time postoperatively. This is ethically acceptable if the tissues are not used for research and are destroyed if the consent is not obtained. The second factor is that time and effort (cost) are spent in obtaining the consent. Unfortunately, some surgical cases may not yield tissue for research, and thus the expense to consent the patient yielded no tissue. The reasons that affect tissue yield are: the tissue may not reflect the diagnosis of interest, which may be determined by frozen section at the time of the surgical procedure; the patient's diagnosis takes precedence, and remainder tissue may not be available for research; or the tissue may not be resected. These determinations can only be made by the appropriate physician (surgeon or pathologist). Therefore, the cost for consent can be reduced when only consenting a patient whose tissue has been collected.

One deterrent to the postcollection consent process is the potential absence of presurgical blood draw or urine collection to pair with the collected tissue. Remnant blood from clinical phlebotomy performed for diagnostic purposes may exist and can be submitted to the biorepository, but it may be suboptimal for any of the following reasons: delayed processing, presence of collection tube additives, insufficient volumes, and unacceptably long time-to-fixation for blood products (eg, access of, aliquoting, and freezing). Blood draws performed for nondiagnostic purposes and *without* prior patient consent for participation in the biorepository are prohibited universally; in the event that blood was drawn under such circumstances, it should be discarded.

Discussing the consent of a patient with their surgeon is important to maintain appropriate physician-to-patient relationships. For this reason, it is ideal to involve surgeons early in the process so that patients can come to surgery already informed and ready to sign the consent. If patients are identified as those previously approached for consent, yet there is no record of confirmation or denial, they can be approached on the day of surgery to finalize the consent process. For some procedures, additional information from the surgeon regarding tumor size, staging, or prior treatment may also help to better define eligibility and avoid the time-consuming practice of obtaining consent from patients who may not have tumors or diseased tissue of sufficient size for banking. Alternatively, all patients who are scheduled for diagnostic blood draws may be approached for consent of whole-blood collection, independent of whether tissue will be placed in the biorepository. Blood collection should be coordinated with other preoperative or postoperative draws. Timing of blood collection may be dependent on the expected use of the blood or blood derivatives. For example, if the blood is primarily being used for germline DNA, preoperative or postoperative blood collection would be acceptable; however, if blood or its by-products were being used for the detection of biomarkers before surgery, then preoperative blood drawing would be required. Furthermore, if blood products are to be used for time-sensitive processing such as for proteomics, the adequacy of pre- or postoperative blood draws should be determined.

The efficiency and universal approach of an informed consent process by institution can be designed to include many individuals, projects, and processes that then coalesce to the focal point of collection, biorepository management, and use. The choice to have an informed consent process as part of the biorepository operations at an institutional level should be based on the inclusion and complexity of research activities of the institution. Regardless of the design chosen, the informed consent and acquisition processes are critical features for the most effective use of the biorepository's management of biospecimens.

Because the informed consent document will indicate for which purposes the collected biospecimens can be used, it is important to thoroughly review and understand the consent elements on downstream research utility. Informed consent written for a specific study, with little latitude in the use of the biospecimens, will limit the use of the biospecimen. For example, checkboxes in the informed consent document, where the patient can check various applied uses, will create a group of biospecimens with variable uses and limit the broad use of the biospecimens in research, not to mention introducing a high degree of complexity in tracking each consent variable for each biospecimen by the biorepository. This is not to say that biospecimen collections should not be collected and managed for specific research projects, but because the informed consent determines the use of the biospecimen, it is recommended that the consent document state that biospecimens may be used for the specific research and undefined future research, thereby reducing the barriers to future research use and supporting the patient's interest in providing a valuable donation (their biospecimen) to contribute to future research findings.

Considerations for genetic research should be directly implied in the consent language, and declarations should be made to ensure the patient's privacy and identity protection. To assist with these assurances, a biorepository can acquire a Certificate of Confidentiality from the NIH and discuss the value of the Genetic Information Nondiscrimination Act, which was designed to prohibit the use of genetic information in health insurance and employment.

Another important document to ensure patient identity protection is a Biorepository Distribution and Use Agreement (BDUA), which is received from the investigator when biospecimens are distributed. This agreement requires the investigator to sign an ethical statement and condition for the use of the biospecimens that states the investigator will not attempt to identify the patient or redistribute the patient's biospecimen. While it is impractical to indicate or guarantee to a patient that their identity could never be breached, it is also impractical to suggest that research systems could ensure that investigators will never improperly manage a biospecimen. Implementation of a BDUA, along with continued education on the conduct of research using human subjects' biospecimens, are effective ways to reduce the potential compromise of patients' privacy/identity.

Biospecimen Collection

Biospecimens can include remnant tissues from surgical resection, body fluids, blood, blood by-products, bone marrow, bronchial alveolar lavage, buccal swabs, hair, fingernails, toenails, and any other approved specimens. Blood and other body fluids can be collected at a variety of points in the clinical process. Whole blood is collected for a variety of purposes, including germline DNA, and for a variety of laboratory analyses that may be done on whole blood or blood fractions, including serum, plasma, and lymphocytes. When possible, phlebotomy for research purposes should occur during scheduled clinical services to minimize additional procedures to the patient; blood draws that are strictly for the biorepository, outside of scheduled clinical services, will carry a higher cost to the biorepository program. Whole blood should be processed to the prescribed derivatives as soon as possible to minimize degradation of the analytes. Processes may include fractionation, cryopreservation, or purification of nucleic acids or proteins. If blood is collected off site and cannot be processed before shipment, it should be maintained at the prescribed temperatures according to a collection protocol. Temperature ranges should also be maintained throughout the shipment process and receipt at the biorepository by means such as insulated shipping kits. A completed chain of custody must also follow the biospecimen from collection to receipt, which includes the important collection and transportation information, such as a biospecimen shipping manifest; the names of personnel collecting, shipping, and receiving the samples; the dates and times at each point in the process; relevant packaging temperature measurements; and courier tracking numbers.

Tissues being transported from surgery to pathology are best managed with a defined notification procedure to the OR team of the intent to collect tissue for research, followed by an expedited transport process to deliver the tissue to pathology immediately after resection, much like a frozen section procedure. The notifications and case management should also ensure that surgically excised tissue is not placed in a fixative upon resection but is maintained in a fresh state for gross dissection and tissue selection for research. The use of a wet-ice bucket is one method to maintain sample integrity to the point of dissection and final fixation (chemical or temperature) of the excised tissue, although if the retrieval process is timely, the extra effort to provide wet ice to and from the OR may not be needed. If processing of the biospecimen is delayed, biological support media or saline solutions (such as Hanks' buffered saline) may be used in conjunction with wet ice to minimize degradation. Best practices suggest a 30-minute limit for the time from excision in the OR to the fixed state (chemical or frozen) as the target for processing tissue.[6] The loss or gain of biological analytes due to the tissue-processing preanalytic variables is still being measured, and at the present time a requirement to snap-freeze tissue in the OR is not supported by the literature. Overall, the collection of biospecimens from the patient to the OR team to the pathology department to the biorepository and finally to the investigator is best managed using well-trained and dedicated research staff. This staff may also be the best group to administer the informed consent because of their familiarity with and understanding of the biorepository.

For institutions just beginning, the tissue delivery from the OR to the pathology department in an expedient fashion for tissue research collections will likely be a new process. New procedures to notify the pathology gross room or frozen section team of consented cases also assist in reducing wasted efforts of the procurement process and postprocurement destruction by the biorepository personnel. Specifically, in the tissue collection procedures, a short delay from tissue banking to distribution that is longer than the diagnostic timeline provides the pathologist with a process if ever there was a need to recall tissue that may be perceived to be useful in aiding the clinical review. (This process has been an experience that has occurred in a few very rare circumstances over many thousands of tissue samples procured by the authors of this chapter.) When tissues cannot be held before distribution—as in the case of cell line development or xenotransplantation—clear communication with the pathologist or pathology assistant (PA) and a practice to collect an extra quality-control sample may be helpful.

Tissue harvesting performed before complete gross examination and sample selection by research tissue procurement personnel, surgeons, and/or surgical residents/fellows must be scrutinized and documented to ensure that the diagnostic tissue is not compromised. When surgical margin evaluation is necessary, the specimen should be inked before being harvested. If tissue is harvested by the surgeon after-hours or at an off-site location without inking of margins, the margin incised to access tissue desired for harvesting should be reapproximated by suture and clearly designated to ensure that the margin is not falsely reported.

The same practices discussed above should be followed for tissue procurement from patients (who have given informed consent) at off-site locations. Standard operating procedures, training, and appropriate documentation of the steps is important so that tissues in the biorepository are not discordant in quality and usability. Off-site extirpation and subsequent specimen transportation to the laboratory should be subject to tracking, shipping, and temperature-monitoring standards established for specimens by the biorepository or other regulatory agencies. Generally, erring on the side of more documentation rather than less, no matter how trivial it may seem, may better enable decisions about the use and disposition of tissue(s), including regarding questions that are related to the patient's health care.

Personnel involved in the sampling and collecting of remnant tissue from surgical resection should be adequately trained in tissue procurement procedures and gross examination. Optimally, the tissue harvesting and subsequent gross examination will be performed by the same individual, providing a seamless transition between research sampling and tissue sampling for diagnosis and staging. Therefore, pathologists, PAs, and residents or fellows in anatomic pathology each must possess the necessary skills to accomplish these tasks. The most critical function is to minimize the risk and prevent compromising tissue diagnosis. However, these individuals are not always available to complete the processing and preparation of the research tissue to its fixed state or to annotate the biospecimen and document the processes. It is recommended that trained procurement personnel assist in the preparation, annotation, and storage of tissue once harvested by the clinical staff. Utilization of laboratory or research assistants/

technicians provides a cost-effective alternative to pathologists, PAs, and residents/fellows and also ensures that the tissue is processed in a complete and timely manner. Pathologists, PAs, and residents/fellows often will be simultaneously involved with triaging the specimen for diagnostic purposes and ancillary studies while harvesting tissue. Dedicated personnel for procurement processes expedite the management of the tissue and reduce the effects of preanalytic variables such as ischemic injury. Laboratory and research assistants/technicians also provide a dedicated pool of personnel to perform procurement tasks with consistency and developed expertise. These personnel may also be intimately involved with IRB approval, forming and writing biorepository and laboratory procedures.

The institution will also need to determine procedures for collection of tissues after normal working hours of the tissue procurement staff. If the appropriate pathology staff is not available, tissue collection may be limited. To decrease the amount of effort needed to complete the tissue processing, tissues can be processed to a desired fixed state, and the follow-up annotation and documentation can be completed by the tissue procurement personnel on the following day. If research tissue procurement personnel are used in substitution of a pathologist, PA, or resident/fellow, proper and precise documentation of tissue sampling is necessary. Such individuals are subject to institutional policies with respect to licensure and accreditation requirements to perform harvesting and procurement. Dimensions, weights, and relationships to relevant margins/structures must be documented and photographed to ensure accuracy of subsequent gross examination.

Tissue harvesting after regular work hours and at off-site surgical centers may complicate or eliminate the role of the pathology laboratory personnel in the procurement process because of logistics and staffing limitations. Trained research tissue procurement personnel, surgeons, and surgical residents/fellows may be utilized in these instances. Off-site surgical sites must be adequately equipped for triaging and procuring tissue in a timely manner. OR personnel must be educated and protocols established to ensure that the procurement of tissue is performed in an expedient manner without compromising tissue integrity and diagnosis. After-hours, off-site, and weekend protocols vary by institution. To obtain all available consented tissue from emergent surgeries, procurement/laboratory personnel or alternate trained personnel may need to be available to procure tissue in a timely manner without compromising diagnosis. This may require flexible work schedules or staggered work shifts to accommodate a surgery schedule that may start early in the morning or run late into the evening. As noted, there are many potential issues in collecting specimens uniformly from site to site, such as consistency of time lines and procedural standards. Variations in the procedures at different collection sites may create additional preanalytic variables that could affect tissue quality. Although it may not be possible to strictly control differences in procedures from site to site, best practices require that procedures be performed similarly, and that is best ensured through training. Moreover, the parameters of the procurement process (eg, cold ischemic time [time to fixation], fixation type, time in fixative, storage temperature, storage duration, transport methods, and transport temperature) should be documented to allow for assessment of the processes that may have an effect on tissue quality. This information can also help in retraining personnel to tighten up variations in collections or in ruling out a collection site from providing biospecimens.

Education and Establishment of Policies for the Collection of Tissues

Education about the procurement of biospecimens and preparation for the process to procure remnant tissue for research is important for pathologists, PAs, residents, fellows, or any other personnel designated to appropriately select remnant tissue, eg, remaining tissue not needed for diagnosis. Although one would expect it to be an inherent part of their professional training, pathologists and PAs generally have not received specific training to appropriately select remnant tissue for research. Research-interest decision points in this process may vary from the traditional training for the submission of tissue for diagnosis. It would be expected that the most acceptable decision points would follow the requirements for the submission of tissue for diagnosis or standard of care; however, decisions to submit tissue for diagnosis can vary, and the need to have tissue that best reflects the research question(s) may drive the consideration to provide remnant tissues for research use. The boundaries of these determinations can sometimes be difficult, and thus discussions between the pathologists and the researcher are helpful to establish what can be provided to advance the research while not compromising the diagnosis of the individual patient. Therefore, it is wise for pathologists to review the requests to provide tissue for research and develop a plan for the procurement of the tissue for research while maintaining the ethical and legal principles of health care to the patient.

Experience has shown that research investigators who do not understand the processes and decision points of anatomic pathology procedures sometimes submit requests for tissue procurement that are not feasible. An early review by the pathologist of the tissue procurement request will more accurately determine what tissues are available and minimize frustrations in the procurement process and research endeavor. Decisions to not collect tissues for a research project should be communicated to the researcher, and if adjustments in the procurement of the target tissue can be made, then the prospects of completion of the research project are improved. Through the project planning analysis, the pathologist can actively educate and aid the research process by estimating the collection timelines that match the research design and setting the appropriate expectation.

Managed appropriately, a biorepository collection for undefined research use can significantly aid in shortening the time to collection for research investigators because pathologists can focus on collecting tissues that will most probably be needed by research investigators at their institution without having an already approved research request in place. Establishment of minimum size thresholds for malignant lesions without previous diagnosis can ensure that researchers and procurement staff do not compromise diagnosis and increase operational costs. Staff and researcher education regarding ancillary testing (eg, chemotherapy resistance assays, cytogenetics, flow cytometry) for specific lesion types can reduce the costs of obtaining consent from patients who may be able to provide fluids but not tissue.

Biospecimen Processing and Quality

Tissue injury associated with prolonged ischemia is a major hurdle for researchers and biorepository personnel.[7] Various studies have shown that RNA degradation and differential gene expression directly correlate with prolonged ischemia.[8] Tissues snap-frozen within as little as 1 hour of extirpation exhibit alterations secondary to RNA degradation. Formalin-fixed paraffin-embedded (FFPE) specimens suffer similar degradation, which is probably secondary to the variable rate of penetration as based on tissue type and size, coupled with the slow rate of fixation by widely used neutral buffered formalin.[7,8] Optimal tissue sample size and environmental pressure can greatly reduce the tissue injury associated with ischemia.[9]

Procurement personnel should have collection materials prepared in advance of acquiring tissue, with sampling containers labeled with an assigned, unique identifier to expedite the processing of tissue upon receipt. Procurement personnel should be readily available to receive harvested tissue from the pathologist, PA, or resident/fellow in an expedient manner to reduce negative effects on the quality of the tissue. Procurement personnel often will further divide remnant tissue and process the aliquots according to investigator and/or biorepository guidelines. A plan to bank the number and amount of the aliquots for tissue and blood should be discussed to meet the design and cost of the biorepository or specific research project. Minimizing future freeze–thaw cycles may require processing the biospecimens into smaller aliquots for storage or the use of new technologies. One method—such as the Frozen Tissue Aliquotter (CryoXtract, Woburn, MA), which removes frozen core aliquots from the original serum or plasma aliquot—allows an original aliquot to be sampled without thawing and refreezing. Generally, 30 mg of cellular tissues will yield sufficient quantities of DNA and RNA for molecular techniques. A larger amount of acellular tissues, such as breast or adipose, will require larger amounts of tissue. In general, the smallest aliquot size for collection and storage of tissue ranges from 100 to 200 mg (relative to density of water this equals 1.0–2.0 mm^3).

For serum or plasma blood products, minimum quantities range from 0.3 mL (in straws) to 0.5 mL (in 1.0-mL cryovials). Urine is usually stored in larger quantities (20 mL or more), primarily because this fluid is often concentrated to increase analyte concentrations. When considering the final volume-to-air ratios in a specimen storage vial, it is a good idea to limit excess air space in cryovials and tubes used for long-term storage of frozen fluids or tissues because this may retard sublimation. Moreover, aliquoting and storing biospecimens in the most efficient manner helps align the costs of a biorepository against excessive banking practices. Documentation data for the biospecimens, as required by the biorepository's protocol, should be captured on data collection forms or electronic data systems at the time of processing and aliquoting.

Tissues should be triaged and processed as quickly as possible to reduce ischemic injury and degradation. Once the tissues have been prepared in a stable preserved or fixed state—whether that involves chemicals (eg, formalin or nucleic acid lysis buffers), cryofreezing, or other preparations—they can be safely transferred to the biorepository for storage. If the biorepository is located at or near the collection site, the transportation of the biospecimens can be as simple as personnel moving the samples from procurement to the biorepository storage; however, in

Table 5-1. Types of Long-Term Storage for Biospecimens

Storage	Specimen
RT (22–25°C)	▪ Formalin-fixed paraffin-embedded (FFPE) tissue
RF (2–8°C)	▪ Fluorescent-stained tissue on microscope slides ▪ Unstained tissue sections on microscope slides
Fz (-20°C)	▪ PAXgene-fixed paraffin-embedded (PFPE) tissue ▪ Isolated/purified DNA
Ufz (-80°C)	▪ OCT-embedded tissue ▪ Isolated/purified RNA ▪ Serum ▪ Plasma ▪ Cerebrospinal fluid ▪ Pleural fluid ▪ Bronchial alveolar lavage ▪ Sputum ▪ Saliva ▪ Urine ▪ Whole blood ▪ Cell pellets
LN_2 (-196°C)	▪ Cryopreserved cells ▪ Snap-frozen tissue

Abbreviations: RT, room temperature; RF, refrigerated; Fz, frozen; Ufz, ultra-low frozen; LN_2, liquid nitrogen.

the event that the biorepository is located at a distant location within the institution or off site, biospecimens must be properly transported. This transport will require packaging of the specimens according to IATA and/or Department of Transportation regulations with proper temperature-regulating materials such as dry ice or freezer packs, as mentioned previously. Chain-of-custody documentation, data collection forms, manifests, and other relevant transportation forms must also accompany the biospecimens throughout the transferal process.

Biospecimen Storage

Many biorepositories have multiple storage types. The types often described are ambient/room temperature (RT; 22–25°C), refrigerated (RF; 2–8°C), frozen (Fz; -20°C), ultra-low frozen (Ufz; -80°C), and liquid nitrogen frozen (LN_2; -196°C). Each biorepository needs to determine the storage types it needs and assign acceptable temperature ranges for each type. Processing protocols should describe the type of long-term storage required for those biospecimens. Table 5-1 provides acceptable storage temperatures of biospecimens on the basis of how they were processed. Stabilization products available to biorepositories, such as for the stabilization of nucleic acids, are not discussed. We encourage readers to continue to review literature on new methods and compounds frequently.

Once received by the biorepository, biospecimens should be placed into proper long-term storage as quickly as possible. It is good practice to document the temperature of biospecimen kits when they arrive at the biorepository (unless temperature data loggers are used). The temperature of the shipping box's inner chambers can be taken upon receipt and recorded along with other sample data for those specimens. The chain-of-custody documentation should be completed and verified for accuracy. Data collection forms are best managed by transcribing or electronic transfer into a biospecimen inventory system along with the final storage location. Barcoded elements can aid in accurately tracking and transferring biospecimens and associated data. This should be a strong consideration in a well-managed biospecimen procurement and biorepository system.

When paraffin-embedded tissue blocks and slides are stored at room temperature, efforts must be made to control humidity, dryness, and insect or rodent pests. Storing unstained tissue sections on slides should be minimized to prevent the loss of antigen integrity. If unstained sections are stored, attempts to protect antigen integrity—such as by storage at refrigerated temperatures with low humidity or by dipping in wax—may provide a degree of downstream use in assays, like immunohistochemistry, for example.[10] Furthermore, water content in tissue is a significant factor for degradation of antigens. Vacuum packing does not prevent degradation of antigenicity if processing does not remove water content in FFPE tissues.[10] Where possible, formalin-fixed tissue specimens should be maintained as paraffin-embedded blocks and sectioned just before staining.

Uniform, evidence-based, biospecimen storage temperatures continue to be determined for biospecimens and derivative analytes. As noted in Table 5-1, at present, -20°C manual-defrost freezers are acceptable for isolated/purified DNA, whereas the ultra-low freezers (-80°C freezers) are recommended for whole blood, cell pellets (for DNA or RNA), plasma, serum, urine, saliva, and isolated RNA. Liquid nitrogen vapor-phase freezers are recommended for tissue and required for cryopreserved cells to develop cell lines. Oxidation and loss of water in frozen tissue are conditions that cause negative changes in antigenicity and morphology, respectively, in biospecimen quality.[11,12] Proper packaging of frozen tissue to reduce access to air and excess humidity in freezers may aid in the reduction of the loss of water through sublimation of an original sample over long storage periods.[13] Multiple thawing and refreezing of frozen biospecimens should also be avoided to minimize damage to proteins and nucleic acids. When thawing–refreezing is necessary, biorepository personnel should record the freeze–thaw cycle numbers in the biorepository informatics database. In the management of biospecimens, it is important to develop an analytical measure of the quality of biospecimens and the stability of analytes of interest. One method of using data loggers included in the shipments provides moment-to-moment temperature data to document the environmental variations to which the biospecimens have been subjected.

Distribution of Biospecimens

When temperature-sensitive tissue is released from the biorepository to distant facilities, temperature stability should be maintained to avoid large variations. Institutions may wish to track shipping vessel temperatures at the times of release and receipt as a quality assurance measure. This can be accomplished through manual temperature measurements or temperature data loggers. Compiled data of temperature fluctuations and spot measures of RNA quality/degradation can provide information to allow the biorepository to adjust practices as necessary. For frozen tissue, packaging on dry ice is the easiest and least costly method to minimize temperature variation for short-term transportation or tissue management. Dry ice has a surface temperature of -78.5°C. Proper containers can maintain frozen temperatures down to -40°C for 48 to 72 hours. Dry ice is the most commonly used temperature management medium for shipments via airlines. The disposal of dry ice is also minimal because of sublimation. Liquid nitrogen has a constant temperature of -196°C and a boiling point of -150°C. It is widely used as a safe method for extreme cold temperature storage, but it requires additional caution during handling and disposal. Liquid nitrogen dry-vapor shipping containers are ideal for maintaining the coldest temperatures to ensure tissue quality and are best for large numbers of cryopreserved cells. Liquid nitrogen dry-vapor shipping containers are expensive to purchase and more expensive to ship compared with shipping kits with dry ice; however, the advantage and justification is that liquid nitrogen offers the coldest temperature for shipment and may be a requirement or preferred choice in the management of specific biospecimens.

FFPE tissue released to distant facilities should be packaged in a manner that prevents exposure to excessive heat. Paraffin wax, depending on the grade, has a melting point ranging from 46°C to 68°C. Although degradation is minimized with adequate fixation, tissue orientation can be compromised within the FFPE block if it is exposed to extreme heat. Freezer packs often are added to insulated shipping containers of FFPE blocks to offset any large, unexpected fluctuations in temperature.

Specimens shipped via ground or air by a commercial carrier must be appropriately packaged and labeled according to international and federal regulations. In general, overnight express delivery services should be used for biospecimens shipped on dry ice or liquid nitrogen. International shipments that would take longer than overnight are possible with attention to increasing the amount of dry ice or coolant, where possible. Express delivery services offer web-based systems to track the route and delivery of a package. The tracking number provides the date of shipment and expected date of delivery to the recipient and allows the clients to track the biospecimens throughout the delivery process. Shipments spanning a weekend should be avoided unless the recipient has verified the ability to accept weekend deliveries. Some specialized couriers will pick up and deliver packages any day or time, but these services will come at a premium price and are generally not the routinely scheduled courier for biorepositories.

Distribution Policies and Procedures for Biospecimens

Biorepositories need to consider appropriate operating procedures in the distribution of biospecimens. To help mitigate issues of patient privacy and ensure that research investigators are aware of the governances in the management of biospecimens, clear policies and documentation for distribution are important. These policies are important because not only are they helpful for present research management, but they may help address future, undetermined guidelines in the use of biospecimens, especially with respect to the discussion about derivatives, such as genetic data, that could be tied to patient identity. An example below, borrowed from the National Cancer Institute's Cooperative Human Tissue Network,[14] and other experiences and sources suggest policies or a distribution agreement would be aligned with the US Department of Health and Human Services Office for Human Research Protections (OHRP) Guidance on Research Involving Coded Private Information or Biological Specimens (http://www.hhs.gov/ohrp/policy/cdebiol.html), which includes the following requirements placed upon the research investigator as a condition for receiving biospecimen materials.

The recipient agrees:

- To not attempt to contact donor patients, treating physicians, or other personnel involved in patient treatment unless prior approval has been granted and the patient has previously consented.
- To not use biospecimens and medical information alone or in conjunction with any other information in an effort to establish the individual identities of patients without specific IRB approval that allows identification.
- To not use the coded biospecimen number supplied in publications.
- To comply with all relevant IRB requirements such that the biospecimens received will be used for the sole purpose described in the approved research project.
- That if the recipient obtains a Material Transfer Agreement (MTA), the agreement is nontransferable and the recipient shall not transfer biospecimens, any portion or derivative thereof, supplied to third parties without the explicit and written permission of the biorepository, and when appropriate, the institution Office of Business Development/Technology Transfer.
- To not sell any portion of the biospecimens provided by the biorepository or products directly extracted from these biospecimens (eg, DNA, RNA, protein), and the recipient will not use the biospecimens directly in a product that is marketed commercially (eg, preparation of control slides), without the prior approval of the biorepository and/or the institution Office of Business Development/Technology Transfer.
- To acknowledge the contributions of the biorepository in all publications resulting from the use of these biospecimens. This would also include recommended wording to be placed in the Materials and Methods or Acknowledgments section, such as, "Biospecimens and associated clinical data were provided by the [institution] and [biorepository name]."

Furthermore, the recipient understands and agrees:

- That although the biorepository attempts to avoid providing biospecimens that are contaminated with highly infectious agents such as hepatitis and HIV, all tissues should be handled as if potentially infectious.
- To acknowledge that the institution where the biospecimens will be used follows Occupational Safety and Health Administration (OSHA) regulations for handling human biospecimens and will instruct their staff to abide by those rules.
- To assume all responsibility for informing and training personnel in the dangers and procedures for safe handling of human biospecimens.
- That when biospecimens are to be used at outside institutions, the institution agrees to be responsible for any claims, costs, and damages or expenses resulting from any injury (including death), damage, or loss that may arise solely from the receipt, handling, storage, and use of biospecimens received from the biorepository to the extent permitted under the laws of this state.

The above text in a document with appropriate signatures is a short track to remind the investigator of his or her obligations (and commitment) to the ethical and legal management of the biospecimen. Depending on the biorepository's institutional governance, many of these statements may be included in its MTA and Data Use Agreement.

References

1. International Air Transport Association. IATA website. http://www.iata.org. Accessed March 31, 2014.
2. United States Department of Transportation website. http://www.dot.gov/. Accessed March 31, 2014.
3. The Genetic Information Nondiscrimination Act of 2008. US Equal Employment Opportunity Commission. http://www.eeoc.gov/laws/statutes/gina.cfm. Accessed March 31, 2014.
4. Office of Extramural Research. National Institutes of Health. Certificates of Confidentiality Kiosk. http://grants.nih.gov/grants/policy/coc/. Accessed March 31, 2014.
5. Hewitt R, Watson PH, Dhir R, et al. Timing of consent for the research use of surgically removed tissue: is post-operative consenting acceptable? *Cancer.* 2009;115(1):4-9.
6. International Society for Biological and Environmental Repositories (ISBER). 2012 best practices for repositories: collection, storage, retrieval and distribution of biological materials for research. *Biopreserv Biobank.* 2012:10(2):79-161. Also available at www.isber.org. Accessed March 31, 2014.
7. Ibberson D, Benes V, Muckenthaler M, Castoldi M. RNA degradation compromises the reliability of microRNA expression profiling. *BMC Biotechnology.* 2009;9:102.
8. Dash A, Maine I, Varambally S, Shen R, Chinnaiyan A, Rubin M. Changes in differential gene expression because of warm ischemia time of radical prostatectomy specimens. *Am J Pathol.* 2002;161(5):1743-1748.

9. Chesnick I, Mason J, O'Leary T, Fowler C. Elevated pressure improves the rate of formalin penetration while preserving tissue morphology. *J Cancer.* 2010;1:178-183.
10. Xie R, Chung J-Y, Ylaya K, et al. Factors influencing the degradation of archival formalin-fixed paraffin-embedded tissue sections. *J Histochem Cytochem.* 2011;59(4):356-365.
11. Engel KB, Moore HM. Effects of preanalytical variables on the detection of proteins by immunohistochemistry in formalin-fixed, paraffin-embedded tissue. *Arch Pathol Lab Med.* 2011:135(5):537-543.
12. Blind C, Koepenik A, Pacyna-Gengelbach M, et al. Antigenicity testing by immunohistochemistry after tissue oxidation. *J Clin Pathol.* 2008;61(1):79-83.
13. Stitt DM, Kastyak-Ibrahim MZ, Liao CR, Morrison J, Albensi BC, Gough KM. Tissue acquisition and storage associated oxidation considerations for FTIR microspectroscopic imaging of polyunsaturated fatty acids. *Vibrational Spectroscopy.* 2012;60:16-22.
14. Cooperative Human Tissue Network. National Cancer Institute. http://chtn.nci.nih.gov/. Accessed March 31, 2014.

Bibliography

Ngapo TM, Babare IH, Reynolds J, Mawson RF. Freezing rate and frozen storage effects on the ultrastructure of samples of pork. *Meat Sci.* 1999;53(3):159-168.

Chapter 6

Quality Control: Providing Useful Specimens to Investigators

Sarah M. Dry
Clara E. Magyar

Background

Most academic medical research centers in this country have a long history of procuring biofluids and human tissues for research purposes. Typically, these were stored in the freezers of individual researchers. Protocols for procurement, storage, databases, and quality control were absent.

The federal government recently became more actively involved in the process of biobanking, spearheaded largely by the National Cancer Institute (NCI). In 2002, the NCI released its first official publication, entitled *Guidelines for Biospecimens* (interactive timeline at http://biospecimens.cancer.gov/about/timeline.asp; contains link to *National Biospecimen Network Blueprint* under 2003). In 2005, the NCI created a biospecimen research unit, initially called the Office of Biorepositories and Biospecimen Research (OBBR), now called the Biorepositories and Biospecimen Research Branch (BBRB). The NCI published *NCI Best Practices for Biospecimen Resources* in 2004, followed by a revised version in 2007, and a new second revision in 2011 (http://www.biospecimens.cancer.gov). The best practice guidelines, released by the NCI, mirror practices at the nation's best-established biorepositories.

The NCI, through the BBRB, has been a vocal advocate for improving biospecimen quality and has encouraged examination of how multiple preprocurement, postprocurement, and biospecimen-processing factors may affect the biological signature of tissues. For example, do specific anesthetic drugs (preprocurement), ischemic times (periprocurement), or length and temperature of storage (postprocurement) affect the expression of DNA, RNA, proteins, and other cellular constituents? How do multiple variables at different stages of the biospecimen procurement process affect these cellular components, and how might this affect research data?

The NCI/OBBR established the Biospecimen Research Network (BRN) in 2006 to understand how different preanalytic variables may affect molecular information derived from biofluids and tissues. The BRN includes several different and complementary efforts, including funding research projects (intramural and extramural) and developing an online, searchable, bioresearch database that lists pertinent publications (http://biospecimens.cancer.gov/researchnetwork/). The BRN also hosts meetings for researchers and biobankers to discuss the latest research data and help identify topics that require additional investigation. Through these efforts, the NCI hopes to identify critical variables during the biospecimen procurement process and develop indicators of quality that are based on research data. The NCI believes this will allow biobankers to optimize their practices in order to provide more uniform and high-quality biosamples for evolving "omics" research platforms and personalized medicine, research, diagnosis, and therapeutics.

The International Society for Biological and Environmental Repositories (ISBER) represents another important voice in the discussion of biorepository practices and biosample quality. ISBER released their third edition of *Best Practices for Repositories* in the April 2012 issue of *Biopreservation and Biobanking (BIO)*. Moreover, ISBER offers a Self-Assessment Tool (SAT) for repositories, which allows for repository operators to determine how well their operation follows the ISBER Best Practices guidelines and helps to identify deficiencies to improve biorepository function and management of samples. ISBER also maintains a proficiency testing program in which samples are sent to the biorepository to assess the accuracy of their quality assurance assays and help identify areas where the biorepository may need to address staff performance or equipment recalibration. The areas for proficiency testing include DNA quantification and purity, RNA integrity, cell viability, tissue histology, and tissue antigenicity. (ISBER Best Practices, SAT, and proficiency test information available at www.isber.org.)

In 2012, the College of American Pathologists (CAP) began a new accreditation program for biorepositories. By the end of 2013, 23 biorepositories had been accredited by the CAP. The CAP standards for biorepositories are unique and were informed by "best practice" recommendations from the NCI and ISBER. Similar to other CAP laboratory accreditation programs, biorepositories need to demonstrate they follow CAP standard practices for biobanking, provide appropriate documentation, and pass CAP inspection in order to receive accreditation. A complete updated laboratory manual is expected. CAP accreditation includes standards for specimen handling, specimen processing (including molecular derivatives, digital image capture, tissue microarray construction, laser capture microdissection, and cell fractionation), instrument and equipment operation, information technology systems, distribution policies, and regulatory issues (informed consent, Institutional Review Board approvals, and Material Transfer Agreements), in addition to basic laboratory standards (safety, training, personnel).[1]

CAP accreditation could have a major impact on the structure and operations of biobanks within the United States. While accreditation is voluntary, this will set a standard for high-quality biobanking operations, and CAP accreditation thus will serve as a surrogate marker for high-quality biosamples. It is not inconceivable that, in the future, CAP or another form of biobank accreditation/certification may be required for grant funding or manuscript publication, as evidence that the research uses high-quality biosamples. Accreditation requires effort to maintain documentation of practices, train staff, and prepare for inspections. Expenses to biobanks for accreditation include direct fees to the CAP of several thousand dollars annually plus personnel time. For all these reasons, CAP accreditation may result in consolidation of biobanks into institutional biorepository resources, unlike the current situation where multiple, separate, individual researcher-controlled freezers hold biosamples. Of note, Canada established a national biorepository network in 2013 and implemented a national accreditation program in 2011 (Canadian Tumor Repository Network, www.ctrnet.ca).[2]

Much more research will be required to develop a full understanding of how biosamples are affected by individual variables and whether all biosamples are affected similarly. For example, existing studies of biofluids indicate variable effects of freeze–thaw cycles on different analytes.[3] It largely remains unclear which variables could make biosamples (tissues and fluids) suboptimal or unsuitable for research. Certain variables may so alter a particular cellular component (for example, prolonged warm ischemia time affects expression levels of phosphorylated proteins) as to make those tissues unsuitable for particular research projects. On the other hand, drug development strategies may seek stable cellular targets, and such research thus may favor tissues associated with a wide range of iatrogenic and physiologic variables. Highly successfully personalized therapeutics (such as Herceptin against HER2) were developed based on research using biosamples that likely were subjected to a wide range of procurement variables. Attention must be paid to the potential effects of procurement variables on biosample quality and downstream testing results. Ongoing research should help identify and clarify factors important to successful research use of biosamples.

This chapter cannot comprehensively address every factor that affects biospecimen quality. Biospecimens constitute a diverse set of human biological fluids and tissues, each with unique biological characteristics. Complicating this natural biological complexity are the numerous specific research questions that may be studied using biospecimens. Ideally, biospecimens should be collected, handled, stored, and tested in a manner that will protect the specific biological components (such as proteins or nucleic acids) being tested in the research study. In reality, many biobanks collect and store biospecimens for future research studies that have not been designed at the time of collection. Specimens banked for future, unspecified research use are often highly valuable because they can be clinically annotated during the course of their "lifetime" with evolving data about the donor. The challenge for biobanks collecting samples for future unidentified research projects is to collect and store biospecimens in a manner that best reflects the original sample and allows the broadest possible research use.

In this chapter we outline strategies that biobanks can use to optimize and standardize their biospecimen procurement, handling, storage, and distribution practices. Biobanks will need to remain aware of emerging recommendations from the BBRB, ISBER, and other organizations, as well as new research findings, and incorporate these into their practices as needed. Excellent resources in this regard are annual meetings of the BBRB and ISBER and their associated websites (biospecimens.cancer.gov, www.isber.org), and other biospecimen-specific websites (eg, Biopreservation Core Resource [BioCoR] at the University of Minnesota, biocor.umn.edu).

Steps That Biobanks Can Take to Optimize the Quality and Usefulness of Stored Specimens

Until more definitive evidence becomes available regarding optimal biospecimen procurement, handling, storage, processing, and distribution practices, specific, universally accepted guidelines may not always be available. Fortunately, resources are available to help biobankers determine if optimal preprocurement, procurement, storage, processing, and distribution variables exist for the samples they intend to procure or for the analytes that will be studied from the sample (ISBER Proficiency Test [www.isber.org], the BBRB Biospecimen Research Database [brd.nci.nih.gov/], the University of Minnesota BioCoR Resources [biocor.umn.edu/biocor-resources]). As noted above, when biobankers know exactly how a sample will be studied, it usually is easier to enact specific, optimal protocols to ensure high biosample quality. When biosamples are being collected for future unspecified use, biobankers can try and determine likely downstream uses for the sample, perhaps by working with researchers, and enact best protocols. For samples where multiple aliquots can be created, biobankers may wish to handle the biosample in more than one way, so as to maximize potential future uses.

There are additional steps that biobanks can adopt that will help standardize the quality of their specimens, may provide data to help researchers select optimal specimens, and will help position the biobank to monitor specimen quality once specific guidelines are issued. These steps involve well-considered, internally consistent procedures and careful documentation of how biospecimens have been handled at every step in the process. When critical variables are documented, researchers will have the option to select or reject biosamples for specific research protocols based on those variables. For example, as noted earlier, phosphorylated protein expression varies considerably during warm ischemia, whereas DNA under the same condition is highly stable. Thus, researcher perception of biosample quality may depend on the variable being studied.

Biobanking operations cannot be entirely automated and will continue to rely heavily on human participation. Thus, biobanking leadership will need to regularly monitor staff performance of quality assurance/quality control (QA/QC) procedures and make adjustments as needed in order to maintain consistently excellent operations.

Identification and Monitoring of Biospecimen Variables

Biobanks must decide to monitor certain variables for all biospecimens. Variables related to procurement, sample processing, storage, and distribution are controlled directly by biobanks and therefore should be handled initially. These are discussed below.

In contrast, preprocurement variables typically involve many departments (eg, anesthesia, surgery, medicine, and oncology) and may not be readily available to biobank personnel. Preprocurement variables include social history (eg, smoking history), regular medications (including over-the-counter medications or herbal remedies), coexistent medical conditions (such as hypertension or diabetes), current treatments that may relate to the biospecimen (such as neoadjuvant chemoradiation), or other specific patient-related variables (such as whether the specimen was obtained in a fasting versus nonfasting state). Pericollection variables for tissues include a broad array of intraoperative variables, such as exact drugs and dosages given by anesthesiologists during surgery, intraoperative blood loss, hemodilution secondary to intraoperative fluid administration, administration of blood or blood products, variation in vital signs during surgery, clamping time for major and minor vasculature, total duration of anesthesia, and duration of intraabdominal insufflation for laparoscopic procedures. Future advances in electronic medical record keeping and institutional middleware information technology solutions may facilitate efforts to obtain these data. Published research data indicates that some of the above mentioned variables (such as medications, fasting versus nonfasting state, hemodilution, duration of intraabdominal insufflation, and anesthesia) do affect analytes and biosamples, but by no means is the list definitive and additional studies need to be performed.[4-6] For other variables (other drugs/dosages, total duration of anesthesia, or use of over-the-counter or herbal remedies), no published data yet exists to indicate that these do or do not affect analytes or biosamples. Individual biobanks will need to determine which of these are not only critical, but measurable, at their institution.

Once biobanks have selected preprocurement, procurement, storage, and distribution variables for tracking, these data should be recorded for each biospecimen. Tracked data can be used for two main purposes. First, the data can be made available to researchers interested in a specific subset of samples to allow them to select those samples best suited for their studies. Second, the biobank can use the data for continual performance improvement. For continual improvement, biobanking leadership must set quality parameters for each variable that they plan to track, analyze this data on a regular basis, and have a plan for how they will investigate and correct their operations when variables fall outside of these parameters. This type of continuous quality improvement is typical in the clinical laboratory setting but has not necessarily been implemented by biobankers. An excellent quality improvement program requires adequate numbers of well-trained staff who reliably follow an organized program of data collection, data interpretation, and investigation. Excellent resources for biobanks seeking to evaluate their existing quality improvement program or develop a new program are available with the ISBER Self-Assesment Tool and through the CAP Biorepository Accreditation Program.

Optimally, the data should be linked to the biospecimen in such a way that biobanking staff or researchers can view the data to determine if the specimen is appropriate for a particular project. This will almost certainly require the use of a sophisticated electronic database (these issues are discussed in detail in chapter 7, *Biorepository Informatics*), unless the biobank is very small. As our understanding of the effects of iatrogenic variables on biospecimens expands, these data may become more and more important to researchers requesting specific specimens.

Finally, pathology and other clinical data greatly contributes to a biospecimen's research value, yet is not typically considered in discussions of biospecimen QA/QC. Patient outcome data, pathology grade, tumor stage, and serum levels of selected markers (eg, prostate specific antigen) significantly increase a sample's translational research value. Advances in information technology should facilitate identification and attachment of this information to specific biospecimens. Biobank managers should regularly review their current practices in this area and determine if they are meeting the needs of their researchers. Automated downloading of these data from other databases, such as from pathology or laboratory information systems, directly into the biospecimen database would be ideal. Interoperability of database software with other hospital and laboratory systems thus will become increasingly important (see chapter 7, *Biorepository Informatics*).

Variables in Procurement, Processing, and Storage

Documentation of the following steps can be done by many biobanks:

- Time of specimen receipt by the biobank
- Time of biospecimen stabilization
- Method of biospecimen stabilization (specific biofluid collection tubes, snap-freezing, formalin fixation, specific media, or other)
- Original volume received and number/size of aliquots
- Method and conditions of separation (if applicable) for biofluids
- Storage (-80°C, liquid nitrogen, or other)
- Any freeze–thaw cycles or significant variations in biosample temperature (number and/or duration of variation with highest/lowest recorded temperature)
- Transport conditions (room temperature, on ice, other) following collection and during distribution/shipping
- Date placed into storage

Other important variables which biobanks may be able to collect include:

- Time from interruption of blood supply (tissues) to final preservation (snap-freezing, formalin fixation, other)
- Time from sample collection (biofluids) to processing/preservation
- Temperature within storage container (continuously or intermittently monitored by thermometers placed at different sites within the storage unit)

There is published research data indicating that many analytes (especially serum or plasma-based analytes) and biosamples are affected by the above variables,[3,7,8] which supports tracking them. Experts agree that the time between biospecimen procurement and stabilization (warm or cold ischemia time) should be as limited as possible, and thus documentation of this variable should be performed if possible. Some information may be difficult to document, especially when the biobank is receiving any type of biosample collected by individuals not directly reporting to the biobank leadership.

We recommend that biobanks develop internal forms to document procurement variables. Internal biobank forms should be simple, ideally with checkboxes. If appropriate, bank accession labels, patient labels, or pathology accession labels can be placed on the forms to eliminate the need to handwrite this information. These approaches facilitate the completion of forms and should remove most objections to their implementation. In our experience, to achieve high-quality data and to receive it consistently, biobank personnel must provide regular performance reports to all individuals involved in biospecimen procurement. Weekly reports by email, with statistics reporting the total number of cases collected and the percentage of cases missing certain variables, are helpful reminders and also generally stimulate improved performance. These reports also can help to identify system-based roadblocks to obtaining certain variables or meeting certain goals. For example, inadequate staffing may result in the warm ischemia time consistently exceeding the bank's target time. Once identified, biobank leadership may be able to find solutions to these types of issues.

If a biospecimen was not collected, we believe it is equally critical for staff to note this and provide an explanation. Again, this can be managed with a checklist for the most common reasons in your biobank, followed by an "other" category. Biofluids and tissues may differ in the most common reasons why specimens are not collected, and forms should be created accordingly. Tissues may not be collected because of insufficient tissue for both diagnostic and research use (the most common reason in our institution), lack of a pathologist or pathology assistant available to release the biospecimen for banking, lack of biorepository staff available to process the tissue, or after-hours arrival. Biofluids may not be collected because of incorrect preparation of the patient (eg, failure to fast after midnight, failure of the patient to arrive, or technical failure [such as multiple failed venipuncture attempts]). Keeping such statistics can be helpful in identifying areas that need additional resources (eg, extending staffing coverage to 9:00 PM rather than 6:00 PM). These statistics are also very helpful in demonstrating biobank capabilities to internal groups or funding agencies, as these data provide explanations for what could erroneously be perceived as suboptimal numbers of cases from which biospecimens have been procured by the bank.

At some point in the biosample process, biobanks must identify and confirm sample composition. This could include pathologic diagnosis and percentage of tumor/normal/necrosis/fibrosis within a tissue sample, and cell viability, tumor content, hemolysis status for a biofluid. Whether this is best performed at or close to the time of procurement or at the time of distribution depends on the individual biobank. This is discussed in detail below ("Quality Control Measures Before Distribution").

Documentation of preprocurement variables presents additional challenges, and biobanks will need to assess the importance and feasibility of obtaining these data. Some variables (such as coexistent medical conditions) may be available to biobank personnel from the electronic medical record; others (such as exact dosages of intraoperative drugs) may require cooperation from other departments. Prior to determining which preprocurement variables to collect, biobanks should communicate with researchers likely to use the samples. If clinical variables already are being collected by another group and are available to the research team, collection by the biobank may not be important. Again, internal forms that track acquisition of this information on each case will be important for biobank leadership to be able to continually evaluate the bank's success in obtaining these variables and in identifying potential solutions if required information is not being obtained routinely.

Quality Control Procedures for Specimen Procurement

All biobanks should have clear, written, standard operating procedures (SOPs) for biospecimen procurement and preservation. CAP accreditation requires a comprehensive laboratory manual with current SOPs for all aspects of the biobank's operations.[9] The biobank's procedures should be reviewed regularly by the biobank director and with biobanking personnel. Additionally, all new staff should be trained in all procedures appropriate to their job description. To ensure procedures are being followed properly, biobank leadership or their designees may review samples collected or directly observe personnel working.

The subsequent paragraphs focus on specific QC procedures for tissue procurement and preservation. Biofluids encompass a broad range of samples, including but not limited to the following: urine, blood, plasma, saliva, cerebrospinal fluid, bronchoalveolar lavage fluid, vaginal secretions, semen, ascites, and stool. Each of these samples requires different procedures for collection, handling, and storage. Even a single biofluid (most obviously blood) may require different handling conditions depending on the analyte to be measured. Proper handling practices for all of these biofluids cannot be adequately addressed in this chapter. However, excellent published references,[10-12] the University of Minnesota consultation services (http://biocor.net/), websites such as the BBRB Biospecimen Research Database (brd.nci.nih.gov/), and biobanking community resources such as ISBER's listserv can provide guidelines and assistance on biofluids or specific analytes within fluids.

A pathologist or a properly trained designee (such as a pathology assistant) must review and select all tissues that will be procured for research. This protects patients by ensuring that adequate tissues remain for diagnostic purposes and that tissues are handled properly, with appropriate attention to surgical margins. Pathologists' medical knowledge, expertise, and experience maximize the selection of appropriate and viable tissues (which is critical for tumors that have received neoadjuvant chemoradiation therapy).

How can one know the actual composition of a tissue sample procured for research? One approach is to create a QC sample for tissues that will be distributed fresh or snap-frozen and banked. Tissue sections for formalin-fixed paraffin-embedded (FFPE) blocks, or for OCT embedding with cryostat sectioning, from one or both sides of the fresh or snap-frozen sample(s) can serve as the QC sections. These sections will be stained with hematoxylin and eosin (H&E) and then interpreted by a pathologist. This H&E slide indicates the composition (ie, diagnosis, tumor relative to normal, percentage necrosis) of the adjacent frozen tissue. Preferably, this slide (or a whole-slide digital image) will be retained permanently. The biobank should determine what information (diagnosis, percent necrosis/fibrosis/tumor) is relevant; ideally, this information will be entered into the biorepository database and readily retrievable in response to biobank or researcher inquiries. The FFPE or OCT blocks have additional research value for immunohistochemistry studies, creating tissue microarrays, or determining gene expression by laser capture microdissection. The timing of creation and evaluation of the QC slide depends on the specific biobank and biospecimen (see "Quality Control Measures Before Distribution" below).

Cross-contamination of tissue samples must be avoided. Current molecular techniques are extremely sensitive, and even relatively few contaminating cells may result in inaccurate data. Optimally, there will be a dedicated area for tissue procurement that is separate from other activities (such as frozen sections or specimen grossing) within the pathology suite. Cutting surfaces should be cleaned between cases, and fresh knife blades should be used between different tissue types—especially tumor versus normal—within the same case. Precautions to minimize RNA degradation, such as wiping cutting surfaces with commercial RNAse removal solutions and keeping specimens on ice, may be considered. Personnel should use personal protective gear during procurement, which also protects tissues from the RNAses ubiquitously present on human skin. If a specimen cannot be attended to immediately, it may be beneficial to place freshly procured tissue into a media such as RNA*later* RNA Stabilization Reagent (Qiagen, Valencia, CA), which has been shown to preserve RNA for molecular studies[13] but have no effect on subsequent processing for histologic or immunochemical analyses.

Sterile tissues may be required for fresh-tissue experiments, such as tissue culture or tumor cell vaccine research. These tissues usually must be procured within the operating room. Once tissues enter the pathology suite, sterility generally cannot be ensured.

Biobank personnel should keep careful track of biosamples procured and/or distributed, thus protecting patients, researchers, and the biorepository. Informed consent language generally gives patients the right to withdraw consent for use of their biosamples in research; in these situations, biosamples that have not yet been distributed will need to be identified and removed from active biorepository storage. Depending on the exact language in the consent, these "recalled" samples may be (1) anonymized and still distributed, (2) destroyed and no longer available for distribution, or (3) retained indefinitely within the biobank. In addition, samples that are banked may sometimes be required for immediate or future diagnostic purposes. A common scenario includes a patient with definite cancer on prostate needle biopsy, but no cancer in the entirely submitted radical prostatectomy specimen. Frozen or formalin-fixed research samples in such cases may be recalled by the attending pathologist for diagnostic purposes. If the pathologist working with the biobank believes it is likely that certain types of samples are at risk for needing to be retrieved from the biobank for diagnostic purposes, it may be wise for the biobank to institute an "embargo" policy for such samples. Embargoed cases are held by the biobank and not distributed for research until the diagnostic report is finalized; this ensures protection of any tissues that may be required for patient care.

Quality Control Measures During Biospecimen Storage

Biobanks must ensure high-quality storage conditions to maintain the highest quality biofluids and tissues possible. As in any clinical laboratory environment, biobanks must have procedures to monitor equipment performance. Secure back-up sources of electricity should be available for all -80°C freezers in the event of a power outage. The biobank should have systems in place, automated or other, to ensure adequate liquid nitrogen levels in storage tanks and a regular supply of liquid nitrogen. Ideally, all -80°C freezers and liquid nitrogen storage tanks should be equipped with automated temperature monitoring and alarm systems to immediately notify staff (via calls, texts, or pages) 24/7 if temperatures exceed the desired range. Staff should visually check the temperatures of all freezers and refrigerators without automated temperature monitoring systems regularly, preferably daily. Written or electronic documentation of freezer/refrigerator temperatures will allow banks to maintain a record of storage conditions, should these be requested by researchers. Any equipment failures should also be documented, including the date, time, duration, and highest temperature recorded. If the temperature failure is severe or prolonged, sample quality may be compromised. In extreme situations, samples may need to be discarded. If specimens are retained, ideally a notation of the equipment failure will be entered into the biobanking database for each sample so that researchers are aware of the potentially compromised sample quality. In the event of equipment or power failures, a sample contingency plan should also be in place to ensure minimal loss of samples, such as sufficient stores of dry ice and availability of back-up freezers for temporary sample storage.

If possible, multiple aliquots of snap-frozen samples from any single procurement or patient should be stored in different freezers. The same practice is recommended for all samples of a particular type (eg, all pancreatic carcinoma samples or all serum samples from a diabetes intervention project). In the event of a freezer failure, this practice will prevent loss of all samples from a particular patient or of a particular sample type.

The duration of tissue formalin fixation affects cellular components and is known to affect certain tests. A well-documented example is the variation in immunohistochemical staining associated with extent of protein cross-linking caused by formalin fixation. For this reason, we recommend that the biobank establish protocols for length of formalin fixation and standardize tissue-processing regimens for these samples.

Any reagents used should be checked regularly. This is especially important for media used to transport fresh specimens, because these media often have short shelf-lives. The expiration date should be written on the side of the container and, for fresh tissue media, should be monitored at least weekly. Each chemical reagent should also have the expiration date clearly written on the container and should be monitored at regular intervals as designated by biorepository leadership.

Documentation of Specimen Quality Measures

As mentioned earlier in this chapter, universally accepted procurement, handling, storage, processing, and distribution practices may not always be available. Similarly, the appropriate QC test to determine sample integrity varies based on the analyte being tested and may not be universally established for a particular sample type. Ideally, a panel of QC tools for samples would be utilized for all possible downstream applications such as genomics, genetics, epigenomics, proteomics, metabolomics, cultures, and xenografts. Currently, this may be unrealistic, because the amount of sample used for QC and the costs associated would diminish the sample available for research and present a significant expense to biobanks and researchers. It is hoped that ongoing research will allow development of appropriate, accurate, and cost-effective QC tests for biospecimens. If the research studies that will be performed on the biospecimen are known at the time of collection, QC tools may be tailored appropriately by biobanking staff. However, this will not apply to biospecimens collected for future, unspecified uses.

In the absence of an ideal test, RNA quantity and quality testing have been used as a surrogate measure of the quality of snap-frozen tissue and biofluids such as blood, plasma, and saliva.[12,14] RNA quality provides an indication of the viability of the tissue at the time of snap-freezing and indicates its suitability for subsequent transcriptomic analyses. Stability of metabolites is also routinely measured in biofluids.[15] Other types of biological fluids may contain a more restricted set of biomolecules (eg, urine because of renal filtration, cerebrospinal fluid because of the blood-brain barrier) and thus require tailored monitoring strategies.[16] Preserving multiple aliquots per sample facilitates quality testing because it will not reduce significantly the samples available for research.

RNA degradation and integrity may be measured with standard gel electrophoresis or by obtaining RNA integrity number (RIN) measurements through RNA electropherograms using systems such as the Agilent 2100 Bioanalyzer (Agilent Technologies, Palo Alto, CA). More recently, microRNA expression profiles (miRNA) in FFPE tissues showed similar profiles to those of fresh tissue and have proven to correlate better than mRNA comparisons.[17] No specific guidelines currently exist regarding the frequency with which RNA QC testing should be performed or the number of samples that should be tested. In addition to monitoring adherence to biobank SOPs for sample procurement and handling, RNA monitoring will allow identification of any problems in the procurement or storage process. Biobanks must be careful in selecting the samples for RNA QC testing. For example, tumors with extensive necrosis (such as glioblastoma multiforme) may show overall low RNA quality and quantity due to tumor necrosis rather than because the samples were procured suboptimally. Biobank leadership should determine what constitutes a representative sampling, both in terms of numbers and types of samples, for their biobank. RNA testing of older frozen samples monitors potential sample degradation during storage. Again, there are no specific guidelines at this time for the number of samples to be tested or the frequency of testing. Testing of older samples can potentially identify malfunctioning freezers. For this reason, testing of a small number of older samples from each freezer used in the biobank may be considered.

If the biobank does not routinely perform RNA testing, arrangements can be made with an appropriately experienced group. Optimally, the testing should be performed under similar conditions by the same group to reduce variations in results due to the testing method itself. Results of this testing should be recorded for each biospecimen and, ideally, be readily accessible to biobanking staff and researchers.

We also ask researchers to share with us their RNA quality and quantity testing results on the specimens we provide to them, thereby increasing the data pertaining to our samples and demonstrating to our researchers our commitment to high quality. If a researcher's results significantly contradict the biobank's overall internal QA/QC performance, this finding should be further investigated. In our experience, this is rare and is more commonly the result of tissue-handling practices by the researcher during RNA testing or the specific RNA extraction techniques being used. In these situations, we first re-review the QC H&E slide that corresponds to the frozen tissue sample in order to confirm that the tissue shows adequate numbers of cells and minimal necrosis. Once reconfirmed, we release a limited number of new samples (usually three to five) as matched aliquots to the researcher and to the laboratory that performs our RNA testing. We ask both laboratories to perform RNA extraction and testing and compare the results.

Quality Control Measures Before Distribution

Proper identification of the sample being distributed remains the most important QC measure at the time of distribution. Staff must cross-check biospecimen labels with the requested sample list. Barcode systems will add an additional level of verification to the process but may not be necessary or cost effective for smaller biobanks.

For tissues, biobanks should verify that characteristics meet those required by the researcher. As noted earlier in this chapter, a useful strategy is to create a matched QC sample for samples that will be snap-frozen and banked or distributed fresh. Tissue sections from one or both sides of the fresh or snap-frozen sample(s) can be formalin fixed and processed and an H&E slide created. A qualified pathologist or designate can evaluate this slide to verify presumed diagnosis, with tumor versus normal tissue usually the most important parameter. Biobanks should determine if additional tissue factors (such as percentage necrosis) will be described for all specimens or only upon request by the researcher. Ideally, the slide will be kept permanently, and the relevant information obtained from the slide will be retained and easily retrievable. Such data may be important if additional aliquots of tissue remain in the bank or if the researcher needs to access this information. The QC slide will also become important if the FFPE block will be used in research, such as for immunohistochemistry studies or for creating tissue microarrays.

Determining when a QC slide should be made and evaluated depends on many factors, including the volume of the biobank, the frequency with which specimens are distributed for research, and the availability of a pathologist to evaluate these tissues. If tissues will be distributed fresh to researchers and used right away, immediate frozen section analysis of the QC sample before tissue distribution may be prudent. If the bank frequently distributes tissues and retains few in storage for any significant period of time, immediate pathologist evaluation of the FFPE QC slide probably is sensible. On the other hand, large procurement operations with a low-to-moderate rate of distribution may find it more efficient to have staff pathologists perform this QC evaluation only prior to tissue distribution.

Quality Control for Equipment and Staff

Biobanks should have procedures for operating, cleaning, calibrating, and changing solutions in equipment/instruments. Biobanks also should maintain a schedule for checking and servicing all equipment and instruments required for their operations, including records of equipment/instrument repair, maintenance, and service. CAP accreditation requires SOPs for all of the above for each piece of equipment/instrument used by the biobank and also requires that instrument repair/maintenance/service records are readily available to all staff and service personnel. As noted above, biobanks should have protocols for temperature monitoring of freezers/refrigerators and a sample contingency plan for freezer/power failure.

Biobank personnel must be properly trained in all biobank procedures for which they are responsible. Biobank leadership and their designees should determine both the elements required for successful performance of each procedure and how competency will be measured. Once determined, biobank leadership will need to determine who will train and evaluate staff on each procedure. Evaluation of competency should be performed on all newly trained staff and on a regular basis (as determined by the biobank director) for existing staff. Training should be documented and these records maintained by the biobank.

Summary

QA/QC processes establish the foundation for an outstanding biobanking operation. QA/QC elements must be considered carefully by biobank leadership before starting a biobank and must be reviewed regularly for existing biobanking operations. If constructed properly, QA/QC programs can help biobank leadership identify deficiencies and continually improve operations. These programs can provide data that will justify requests for additional institutional or grant funding for biobanking operations.

The NCI and ISBER raised awareness of the numerous preprocurement, procurement, storage, and distribution variables that may affect the biological integrity of a biospecimen. We remain in the early stages of fully understanding the impact of these variables on biospecimens and how such variables may affect the suitability of biospecimens for specific types of research. Biobanking leadership should remain aware of updated recommendations from the NCI and ISBER regarding biospecimen quality. The new CAP voluntary Biorepository Accreditation Program sets standards for quality biobanking operations within the United States. This program probably will have a major impact on the structure and operations of biobanks within the US. Biobanks should remain aware of any impact CAP accreditation may have on grant funding for use of biosamples and be aware of any journal criteria for reporting research using biosamples.

Biobanks can and should establish internal goals for biospecimen collection, processing, storage, and distribution. These steps should involve well-considered procedures and careful documentation of how biospecimens have been handled at every step in the process. Biobanking leadership should regularly monitor staff performance of QA/QC procedures and make adjustments as needed in order to maintain consistently excellent operations. In this way, biobanks will be able to standardize the quality of their specimens and help position the biobank to monitor specimen quality when specific guidelines are established.

References

1. CAP Accreditation Program. *Biorepository Checklist: Master.* Northfield, IL: College of American Pathologists; April 2014.
2. Canadian Tumor Repository Network. *Biobank Certification: Development of a Program By the Canadian Tumour Repository Network (CTRNet).* http://biospecimens.cancer.gov/meeting/brnsymposium/2011/Posters/Suggitt-508.pdf. Accessed March 31, 2014.
3. Betsou F, Gunter E, Clements J, et al. Identification of evidence-based biospecimen quality-control tools: a report of the International Society for Biological and Environmental Repositories (ISBER) Biospecimen Science Working Group. *J Mol Diagn.* 2013;15(1):3-16.
4. Schlomm T, Nakel E, Lubke A, et al. Marked gene transcript level alterations occur early during radical prostatectomy. *Eur Urol.* 2008;53(2):333-344.
5. Braz MG, Braz LG, Mazoti MA, et al. Lower levels of DNA damage and apoptosis in lymphocytes from patients undergoing surgery with propofol anesthesia. *Environ Mol Mutagen.* 2012:53(1):70-77.
6. Tu KL, Kaye SB, Sidaras G, Taylor W, Shenkin A. Effect of intraocular surgery and ketamine on aqueous and serum cytokines. *Mol Vis.* 2007:13:1130-1137.
7. Hubel A, Aksan A, Skubiz APN, et al. State of the art in preservation of fluid biospecimens. *Biopreserv Biobank.* 2011;9:237-244.
8. Unhale S, Solomon R, Skubitz APN, Hubel A. Stabilization of tissue specimens for pathological examination and biomedical research. *Biopreserv Biobank.* 2012;10(6):493-500.
9. CAP Accreditation Program. *Biorepository Accreditation Program Checklist: Sample Pages.* Northfield, IL: College of American Pathologists. http://www.cap.org/apps/docs/laboratory_accreditation/lap_info/biorepository_accreditation_program_checklist_sample.pdf. Accessed March 31, 2014.
10. Fowke KR, Behnke J, Hanson C, Shea K, Cosentino LM. Apoptosis: a method for evaluating the cryopreservation of whole blood and peripheral blood mononuclear cells. *J Immunol Methods.* 2000;244(1-2):139-144.
11. Hanna J, Hubel A. Preservation of stem cells. *Organogenesis.* 2009;5(3):134-137.
12. Ugolini D, Neri M, Canessa PA, et al. The CREST biorepository: a tool for molecular epidemiology and translational studies on malignant mesothelioma, lung cancer, and other respiratory tract diseases. *Cancer Epidemiol Biomarkers Prev.* 2008;17(11):3013-3019.
13. Florell SR, Coffin CM, Holden JA, et al. Preservation of RNA for functional genomic studies: a multidisciplinary tumor bank protocol. *Mod Pathol.* 2001;14(2):116-128.
14. Leidinger P, Keller A, Borries A, et al. High-throughput miRNA profiling of human melanoma blood samples. *BMC Cancer.* 2010;10:262.

15. Betsou F, Barnes R, Burke T, et al; for the International Society for Biological and Environmental Repositories (ISBER) Working Group on Biospecimen Science. Human biospecimen research: experimental protocol and quality control tools. *Cancer Epidemiol Biomarkers Prev.* 2009;18(4):1017-1025.
16. Saude EJ, Sykes BD. Urine stability for metabolomic studies: effects of preparation and storage. *Metabolomics.* 2007;3:19-27.
17. Liu A, Tetzlaff MT, Vanbelle P, et al. MicroRNA expression profiling outperforms mRNA expression profiling in formalin-fixed paraffin-embedded tissues. *Int J Clin Exp Pathol.* 2009;2(6):519-527.

Chapter 7

Biorepository Informatics

Mark A. Watson
Rakesh Nagarajan

Biospecimen annotation data may often be as valuable as the biospecimens themselves. Therefore, proper consideration of a data structure and software application to manage biospecimen data is as important as considering proper biospecimen storage and processing procedures. This chapter outlines the key elements of best practices for biorepository informatics, from both a data model and an operational perspective, based on published guidelines[1-3] and user experiences.

System Design

When establishing a biorepository informatics system, the first decision is often whether to build a system "from scratch" or purchase a software application from a commercial vendor. Each approach has its relative advantages. For large, enterprise-scale repositories with little resources for software development, the purchase of a commercial system may be appropriate. Vendor solutions, although sometimes very expensive, provide "out-of-the-box" software applications and, for a price, user training and ongoing software support. However, local data management resources (eg, information technology support) are usually still required to maintain a system (for data back-ups, local system failures, etc) unless a remote hosting solution is chosen. A remotely hosted system, where data is maintained and managed off-site, may not be permissible at some institutions because of Health Insurance Portability and Accountability Act of 1996 (HIPAA) and data privacy issues. The data model and functionality of commercial systems are usually fully vetted by domain experts, and the software, generally developed under best practices of software design, is fully tested. In some cases, however, the design of a commercial software product may be incompatible with or constrain existing repository operations, and although the vendor may be able to provide site-specific modifications to their application, this comes at an added cost.

For these reasons, many repositories elect to develop their own systems for biospecimen data management. Such systems range from ad hoc spreadsheet files to elaborate server-based relational database management systems. A key advantage of independent design is that it allows for the development of a system that is uniquely tailored to each biorepository and at a seemingly low cost relative to purchasing a commercial product. However, building a custom application (beyond the use of a simple spreadsheet application) requires a dedicated team of software designers who understand both the workflow and data management issues in the repository as well as the principles and practices of good software design.[4] Documentation of the development process and detailed user and technical guides are essential components of any locally designed application, which will allow continued use and development long after the original software development team has disbanded. Because it is often difficult to find and fund expert software development personnel on a temporary basis, repositories may elect to outsource software development projects to a commercial entity on a fee-for-service basis. This has the combined advantage of creating a custom application that is designed and documented by professional software developers. A related approach is to utilize an existing, open-source application that can then be further customized for the repository's specific needs. Open-source software is usually free or low cost. Depending upon the software design, it may also be readily amenable to customizations by an institutional or contracted software support team. The National Cancer Institute (NCI)-funded caTissue application is one example of a freely available, open-source software solution for biospecimen informatics.[5]

If a repository elects to design its own informatics solution, there are several design principles that should be followed.[3,4] Initially, the repository director and staff should accurately and comprehensively describe the scope of operations associated with the data that needs to be captured. For example, will the system only be responsible for freezer inventory management? Does the system need to receive and track requests for prospective biospecimen procurement

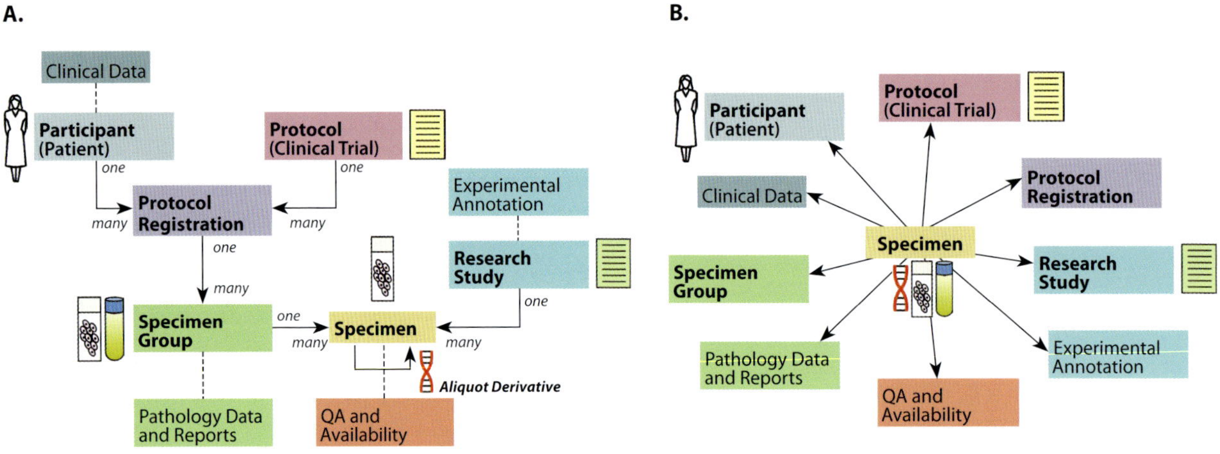

C.

Last Name	First Name	Protocol Title	Registration ID	Specimen Group Name	Specimen Type	Specimen ID
A	B	XYZ	123	Screening	Serum	S001
A	B	XYZ	123	Screening	Saliva	S002
A	B	XYZ	123	Post Therapy	Serum	S003
A	B	XYZ	123	Post Therapy	Saliva	S004
A	B	QRS	456	Screening	Serum	S005
A	B	QRS	456	Post Therapy	Serum	S006
A	B	QRS	456	Post Therapy	Saliva	S007
C	D	XYZ	789	Screening	Serum	S008
C	D	XYZ	789	Screening	Saliva	S009
C	D	XYZ	789	Post Therapy	Serum	S010
C	D	XYZ	789	Post Therapy	Saliva	S011
C	D	QRS	910	Screening	Serum	S012
C	D	QRS	910	Post Therapy	Serum	S013
C	D	QRS	910	Post Therapy	Saliva	S014

D.

Last Name	First Name	Protocol Title	Registration ID	Screening Serum	Screening Saliva	Post Therapy Serum	Post Therapy Saliva
A	B	XYZ	123	S001	S002	S003	S004
A	B	QRS	456	S005	—	S006	S007
C	D	XYZ	789	S008	S009	S010	S011
C	D	QRS	910	S012	—	S013	S014

Figure 7-1. Example of a high-level data model illustrating data classes (ie, data tables), class attributes (ie, data table elements), and "one-to-many" class relationships that might be typically included in a biospecimen informatics system. A, The data model organizes data classes ("participant," "protocol," "specimen," etc) into the most efficient (normalized) hierarchical representation to preserve data integrity. B, Star schema representation of the same data is less efficient (denormalized), although it sometimes allows for simplification and improved performance of complex data queries. In comparison, in nonrelational data schemas such as "flat files" or spreadsheets (C, D), data must often be duplicated for multiple rows (data records) or cross-tabulated in a format that may be inconsistent across data records, difficult for query tasks, and nonextensible as the data set grows in size and complexity.
Abbreviation: QA, quality assurance.

and project management? What types of biospecimens (eg, fresh/frozen tissues, biofluids, archived paraffin tissue blocks, nucleic acid samples) will be tracked by the system? Should the system provide a method for pathologic and clinical annotation of biospecimens? What interfaces need to be provided for searching and reporting data? Will different types of users need different access or views of the data? Will the system need to support shipping and tracking of biospecimens to other institutions? Will the system need to support multiple repositories within an institution? Will the system need to interface with other existing data systems, such as clinical data management systems (CDMS), clinical data warehouses, and systems that manage genomic and other assay data? Once the scope of operations is defined, more specific "use cases" and requirements can be elaborated, which will drive the design approach.

An important concept in either choosing or designing a biospecimen informatics system is to understand the difference but relatedness of the user interface versus the underlying object or data model (Figure 7-1). The user interface of an application defines how all users (biobank staff, investigators, and administrators) enter and view data in the system, including the workflows associated with biospecimen processing and coincident data entry, whereas the model describes how the data is most efficiently and unambiguously represented in the database for search and reporting purposes. The system should allow for convenient and rapid data entry that is intuitive for the end user. Data entry screens and data fields should be arranged and presented in a manner that is most compatible with workflows in the laboratory. For example, if biospecimens are received and processed at an accessioning bench, the system should provide a simple interface to simultaneously enter biospecimen data on many specimens from many individuals at once. When multiple, different workflows are employed in the repository, it can be challenging to design such an all-purpose interface. On the other hand, some perceived convenience features of the user interface—such as the ability to add free-text comments or ad hoc data elements as needed, or the lack of mandatory data fields (such as dates)—can compromise the integrity of the data and/or data model itself.

The selection of a specific database platform (eg, Oracle, MySQL) and programming platform on which to build an informatics system is less critical than the system design itself. Smaller, self-contained biorepositories may build a sufficiently comprehensive system using a desktop or client/server database software application (eg, Access, Filemaker, 4D). Larger, enterprise-scale repositories (particularly those that require data input and retrieval from a wide variety of remote locations) may elect to build a web-based, n-tiered system that includes a relational database layer, an application layer that contains all the business logic and web pages and that interacts with the database layer, and the standard web browser application on the client that can interact with the application layer through appropriate internet connectivity.

Most software design projects employ an iterative approach, which allows for the gradual evolution of the software through multiple prerelease versions that can be fully vetted and tested by end users before the final release. This approach ensures that the final product meets the exact needs and specifications of end users and also allows end users to develop familiarity with the final product before it is put into full production. As noted above, it is important that the release of the application is accompanied by the appropriate design, technical, and end user documentation to ensure that the system can be supported and modified as necessary, well beyond the initial release period.

Data Elements

The types of data and the object model utilized by a repository informatics system will depend upon its scope of operation. Figure 7-1 illustrates one example of an object model. Classes, attributes, permissible values, and the relationships between different classes are important aspects of the model. *Classes* define the physical objects that are tracked in the system, such as patients, biospecimens, and storage locations. *Attributes* are the qualitative or quantitative characteristics of the class or object, such as a patient's gender, the anatomic source of a biospecimen, or the physical location of a freezer. *Permissible values* are constrained values or vocabulary terms that can be assigned to a particular attribute, such as "male" or "female" for patient sex; or "spleen," "liver," or "bone marrow" for a biospecimen anatomic source. Figure 7-2 shows some typical classes and attributes often tracked in a biorepository informatics system. These are briefly discussed below.

Participants and Protocols

In many repositories, biospecimens will be collected as part of an organized research activity. This may be a generalized tissue banking protocol or a highly defined clinical trial. In all cases, collected biospecimens are derived from participants, and those participants are associated with protocols. Therefore, it is important for a biospecimen informatics system to at least represent participants from whom biospecimens are collected and the associated collection activity or protocol in which they are enrolled (Figure 7-1). Even if the intended scope of a biorepository informatics system does not include clinical data, it is often useful to collect key demographic parameters of participants, such as sex and race, for reporting purposes. If the participant's date of birth is captured, then "participant age at collection" can be derived from the participant's birth date and the date of biospecimen collection (recorded as specimen or event data). Otherwise, a dedicated data element for "participant age at collection" is often useful for generating summary demographic reports. In cases where storage of protected health information (PHI) is not permissible, tracking a participant's first and last name initials (which are sometimes physically attached to received specimens) can be useful as a secondary biospecimen identity check. In an environment where the biorepository system can hold PHI (eg, participant's full name, date of birth, medical record number, or other unique identifying information), the information can be stored to unambiguously associate biospecimens collected at different times, locations, or under different protocols to the same individual. The biorepository informatics system should be flexible enough to uniquely identify participants and their biospecimens using both identified and de-identified schemas. The following general information about the collection protocol itself is often useful for administrative purposes: title, activation date, expected accrual (if applicable), and name of investigator. For repositories that are involved in tracking biospecimens from clinical studies or therapeutic trials, it may also be important to represent the registration of a single individual across different trial protocols. Furthermore, trials often collect biospecimens (blood specimens or tumor tissue biopsies) across multiple treatment points in the protocol, and therefore it may be desirable for the biospecimen informatics system to associate groups of specimens within specific time points or study calendar events within a protocol. For pharmacology studies, time points may be measured in minutes, whereas for other clinical trials or studies, they may be far less definitive, such as, "pretherapy," "remission," or "relapse."

Specimens

The most obvious focus of any biorepository informatics system is the biospecimen itself. Depending upon its scope of operations, a biorepository may need to store data about multiple types of speci-

Class	Attribute	Comment / Possible Value Domains
Participant	Last Name First Name Date of Birth Sex Race Vital Status	Some repositories may not collect protected health information (PHI)
Protocol	Title ID Activation Date End Date Projected Accrual	
Protocol Registration	Registration ID Registration Date Age at Registration	
Specimen Group	Collection Time Point Clinical Diagnosis Collection Site Surgical Pathology Case Number	*Screening, Pre-RX, Post-RX, Remission, Relapse, etc* *SNOMED-CT, etc* (May reference a table of institution locations) (For specimens collected during a clinical procedure)
Specimen	Specimen ID Collection Date-Time Stamp Biophysical Type Pathologic Class Pathologic Diagnosis Percentage Tumor Cellularity Anatomic Source Preservation Type Collected Quantity Receipt Quality Available Quantity Storage Location	 *Tissue, Cells, RNA, DNA, Serum, Blood, etc* *Malignant, Premalignant, Metastatic, Healthy, etc* *SNOMED-CT, ICD-O, etc.* (For tumor tissue specimens) *FMA, ICD-O* *Frozen, Cryopreserved, Fixed, etc* (Units dependent on biophysical type) *Adequate, Thawed, Lysed, QNS, etc* (Units dependent on biophysical type)
Study	Study Title Principal Investigator Activation Date End Date IRB Approval Number Distributed Specimens Publications	 (May reference a table of users) (Reference to a table of specimen IDs) (Reference to a table of PubMed IDs)

Figure 7-2. Example of a minimal core set of data classes, attributes, and value domains that may be used by a biorepository tracking system. Additional attributes and classes not listed here may be extended from such a core set of data elements, depending upon the specific needs of the biorepository or the collection protocol for specifying additional information related to participants, biospecimens, biospecimen processing, quality assurance, and assay procedures.

Abbreviations: FMA, Foundation Model of Anatomy Ontology; ICD-O, International Classification of Diseases for Oncology; QNS, quantity not sufficient; IRB, Institutional Review Board.

mens (such as fluids, tissues, cells, nucleic acids), and each of these specimen types may be associated with unique data elements. For example, concentration is a relevant attribute for nucleic acids, but section thickness is relevant for tissue slides. For this reason, each biospecimen type may be represented by a specialized data class that holds attributes or data elements specific for that specimen type. Depending upon the repository's needs, the protocols that it serves, and the underlying data model, it should be possible to associate groups of specimens with specific trial protocols or collection time points. For example, it may be desirable to track the bone marrow samples collected from a single patient before therapy, after therapy, or at relapse that are associated with the patient's enrollment in one or more specific trials or protocols (Figure 7-1). Furthermore, in most repositories, one sample can be processed into multiple other specimens, sometimes of a different specimen type; for example, a tube of whole blood may be spun into plasma and a buffy coat. The spun plasma and buffy coat may be divided and frozen as multiple specimen aliquots. One aliquot of buffy coat may be used for RNA extraction, a second aliquot may be used for DNA extraction, and a final aliquot may be used for a second RNA extraction, several years later. A biorepository informatics system should be able to represent relationships between "parent" and "child" specimens so that, for example, it is possible to identify a DNA preparation that originates from the same paraffin tissue block as a tissue punch used for a particular tissue microarray spot.

Processing Events

Some attributes of a biospecimen are intrinsic and constant to its character (such as its biophysical form or anatomic source). However, other properties of a biospecimen are the result of some event that it experiences as a result of a standard operating procedure for specimen processing, such as collection, centrifugation, freezing, fixation, thawing, transport, distribution, quality review, and so forth. Just as an individual may have a resumé that summarizes his or her life experiences, a biospecimen may have its own "resumé" or "life cycle" that summarizes the processing events that define its character.[6,7] These events may be numerous, repetitive, and varied among individual specimens. Therefore, for maximum flexibility, a biorepository informatics system may track a specimen's life cycle events as individual pieces of data and provide a user interface to search for or report specific life cycle events. However, for simplicity, it may be easier to represent a limited number of key, singular, specimen life cycle events as specific specimen attributes. For example, in the first approach, "warm ischemia time" could be calculated from the duration between a "collection" specimen life cycle event and a "freeze" specimen life cycle event. In the second approach, the data element "warm ischemia time" may just be an attribute of all specimens.

Inventory and Transport

Accurate inventory data is paramount for any biorepository. A fully functioning system should provide real-time accounting of specimen availability and location. Different repositories and different specimen types within a single repository may utilize containers with many different configurations, so the inventory system should have a flexible design. This system could range from a single filing cabinet in which paraffin tissue blocks are stored with no defined internal position to freezer systems where specimen vials are stored within canes or boxes that are part of a highly defined hierarchy of containers. For auditing purposes, the movement of a specimen from one location to another should be tracked (date, time, and user), and the system should provide a simple user interface to record transfers, either at the specimen or entire specimen container level. For regulatory purposes, containers themselves (particularly freezers) may have data collected regarding daily temperature recordings, power outage or unit failure events, and maintenance schedules. In addition to storage position and conditions, the available quantity of a specimen should also be recorded. Although the amount of a specimen may be easy to quantify for fluid, slides, or nucleic acid biospecimens, a more qualitative descriptor may be required for tissue blocks. It may also be desirable to record not only the physical available quantity of a specimen, but also whether a particular specimen is physically available but embargoed on the basis of its pending or potential allocation for a previous request or study.

Quality Assurance

For regulatory purposes, a biorepository may need to record and report several types of quality control parameters. An informatics system should be capable of tracking these parameters. As discussed above, quality assurance data elements may be represented as single attributes of specimens (such as the receipt quality of a blood specimen or the A260:A280 ratio of a nucleic acid specimen) or as multiple recurring "review events" experienced by a specimen over time (such as an RNA sample that is assessed for integrity at the time it is created and then again several years later when it is retrieved from the freezer for secondary use). Specific quality control parameters may vary with a repository's scope of operations and the specimen types that it processes, but they generally include measures of receipt quality (frozen, thawed, inadequate quantity, damaged), physical quality of biofluids (hemolyzed, lipemic), histopathologic quality of tissues (percent tumor cellularity and necrosis), and molecular quality of nucleic acids.

Consent

Depending upon the operations of the repository, it may be desirable or even essential to track patient consent associated with collected biospecimens. Generally, consent for biospecimen research use is defined at the level of the protocol, trial, or collection activity, and one or more specific uses for biospecimens (eg, use for disease-specific research, use for non–disease-specific research, use for genomics research) may be stipulated by each patient. Although this may be uniform for a repository that is involved in a singular collection activity, it is more likely that consent and permissions for research use may vary widely among biospecimens stored in a single facility. In order to ensure that biospecimens are distributed and utilized for research studies that are commensurate with the consent provided by the participant, at a minimum a biorepository informatics system should be able to summarize and report on use permissions for each specimen that is distributed for research. More advanced systems may also implement logic to control or monitor the distribution of specimens to only certain research studies on the basis of the level of informed consent.

Clinical and Pathology Data Annotation

In most cases, biorepository informatics systems do not record detailed clinical data. As noted above, a common set of demographic data (patient sex, race, age at collection, clinical diagnosis) and basic pathology data (histopathologic diagnosis, anatomic sublocation) may be immediately useful for reporting on general specimen availability. Other data may be useful and directly relevant to biospecimen selection for secondary-use research projects but may be more disease or protocol specific. For example, for cancer specimens, tumor TNM stage and grade are useful for specimen selection. For lung cancer, the presence or absence of a smoking history may be important for study design; whereas for breast cancer cases, clinical tumor biomarkers such as estrogen receptor and HER2 receptor status may be important data elements. If not captured within a study time-point or calendar event structure that is part of a more formalized therapeutic trial, it may also be relevant to record information about systematic treatments or exposures experienced by the participant relative to the time of biospecimen collection, because this may modify the biological character of the biospecimen itself (eg, preoperative radiotherapy to tumor tissue may induce significant necrosis in the surgically resected specimen that is collected for the repository). A flexible data schema and user interface that can allow user-defined and protocol- or collection-specific clinical and pathology data annotation may be highly desirable. Alternatively, some biorepository informatics systems may integrate tightly with a parallel CDMS, such that specific patients, protocols/collection efforts, specimen groups, and specimens map directly to clinical data represented in the CDMS for both searching and reporting purposes (Figure 7-3). This approach, however, requires well-integrated systems or a larger (usually commercial) software suite.

Experimental Annotation

Most biorepository systems will only track information about biospecimens themselves. More sophisticated systems may also track experimental annotation on biospecimens, to the extent that it could be useful for selecting specimens for subsequent research studies. For example, a biorepository may wish to capture hormone and growth factor receptor status (performed either in a research setting or clinical laboratory) from breast cancer tumor specimens to aid in the selection of specimens for a future study based on molecular phenotyping. Some repositories may perform whole-slide scanning of stained reference slides from tissue specimens, and, even if the images are not stored within the repository system itself, linkage of the specimen data to the location of the scanned image file can be very useful in reviewing specimens for quality assurance (QA) or study selection purposes. Similarly, investigators may be interested in obtaining banked specimens that have been used previously for the generation of "omics" data, such as microarray-based gene expression profiling or exome sequencing, to leverage previously generated data (either published or not) for their own studies. Like whole-slide scanned images, such data is often too voluminous to be held and managed within the biorepository data system itself, but biospecimen data may include references to the location of one or more data sets that have been previously generated using the specimen.

There are three major challenges in attempting to assign experimental annotation to banked biospecimens. First, there is a need for an efficient mechanism to retrieve experimental data, often from numerous assays performed in many different laboratories. Second, there must be a uniform approach

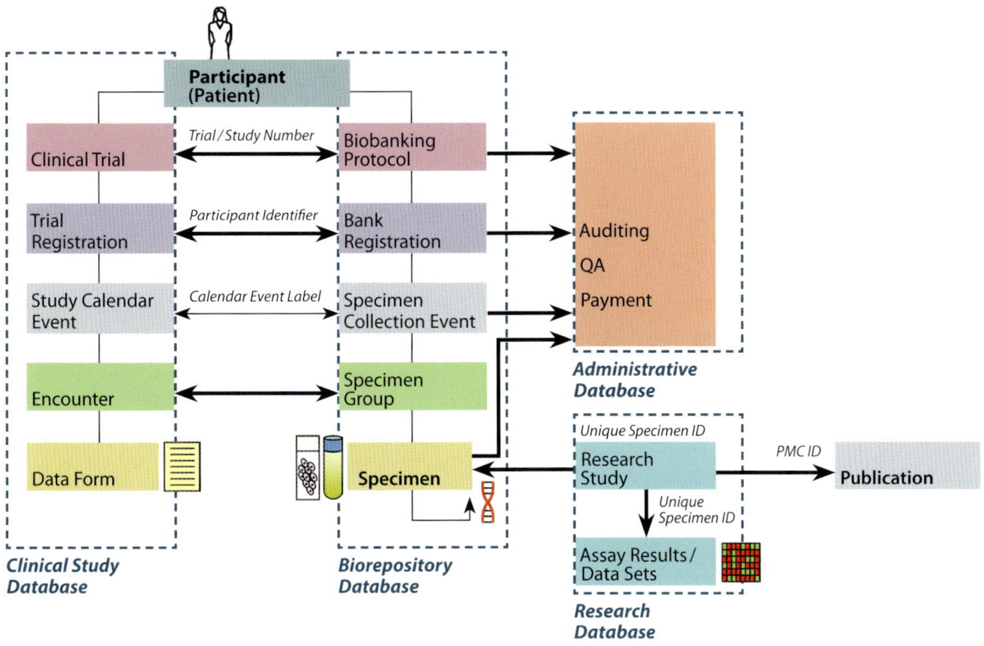

Figure 7-3. Potential integration points between data classes in a biospecimen tracking system and other clinical data or experimental research databases. Links and object (class) identifiers that may be comparable across systems and utilized to build queries across databases are indicated and highlighted by bold arrows. Abbreviations: PMC, PubMed Central; QA, quality assurance.

to expressing diverse sets of experimental assay data (gene sequence, gene expression, protein biomarker) so that they can be easily and intuitively made the subject of any data search. Third, the provenance and QA measures of any experimental assay data should be captured in addition to the actual data. At least in some cases, these challenges can be met when biorepository specimen tracking systems can be programmatically linked or integrated with assay data generated in institution-based core laboratories, such as in a pathology/immunohistochemistry or genomics core laboratory (Figure 7-3).

Requests, Utilization, and Productivity

The value of almost any biorepository is based upon its utilization and contribution to scientific productivity. Therefore, it is important for any biospecimen informatics system to track requests, utilization, and, to the extent possible, scientific productivity. In fact, nearly all of the functioning components of a prospective tissue requisition and procurement service (as opposed to an archival biospecimen repository) may be focused on request and project tracking. At a minimum, the system should record specimen distribution information: to whom, for what project, and when. Specimens collected from multiple sources, sites, or protocols may be distributed for a single research project, so a "many-to-one" relationship between these data classes is required (Figure 7-1). More sophisticated systems may record additional information (if it is obtainable) often needed for annual progress reports, including extramural funding sources for the project, Institutional Review Board (IRB) approvals, and resulting scientific publications. Additional features may allow investigators to search for and immediately request specific banked biospecimens or to submit requests electronically based on more generic biospecimen needs.

Class Relationships

As shown in Figure 7-1, each of the biospecimen data classes described above, as well as potentially several others not enumerated here, should be appropriately associated with each other in the data model. The ability to form "one-to-many," "many-to-one," and "many-to-many" relationships, as well as self associations between data classes, is a significant benefit of employing a relational database management system as opposed to the use of individual "flat files" or spreadsheets. As described above, a single individual may be enrolled in multiple trials or protocols that involve biospecimen collection (one-to-many). A participant enrollee in a trial may contribute specimens at multiple time points in a trial (one-to-many), and each time point may involve the collection of several different specimen types (one-to-many).

A single specimen may be used to derive multiple specimens (one-to-many), and a research study may utilize specimens from more than one patient, protocol, or time period (many-to-one). Although some of these relationships between individuals, protocols, and biospecimens may be coded for within specimen labels themselves (see below), any mislabeling event could lead to a permanent break of this linkage if it is not also properly represented in the data model.

Vocabularies

"The nice thing about standards is that there are so many of them to choose from" is a lament commonly heard in the bioinformatics community. However, given this fact, any biorepository informatics system, either purchased or developed, should aim to use controlled, documented, and appropriately vetted vocabulary terms. This is preferable to the use of ad hoc controlled vocabularies or, even worse, free-text. For example, a tissue specimen that has been fixed in neutral buffered formalin and embedded in paraffin wax may be referred to using many different terms: *paraffin block, fixed tissue, FFPE (formalin-fixed paraffin-embedded), surgical pathology block, embedded tissue,* or *archival tissue.* When any (or all) of these terms is used to describe a single concept in the biorepository database, it may be very difficult to search, track, or report on the availability of all tissues that have been fixed in neutral buffered formalin and embedded in paraffin wax.

Similar problems arise when breast tumor specimens are variously annotated with clinical diagnosis terms such as *invasive ductal carcinoma, breast cancer, infiltrating duct carcinoma, carcinoma of the breast, breast adenocarcinoma,* and so forth. At a more fundamental level, even the understood definition of a data concept such as "specimen" can be ambiguous. For example, if 100 colon cancer tumor "specimens" are available for a research project, does this mean 20 tissue sections obtained from 5 tissue blocks from 1 patient, or 5 tissue sections obtained from a single tissue block from 20 patients, or 1 tissue section obtained from 1 block from each of 100 patients? Although it may not be possible to reach complete consensus on vocabularies across all biorepository and biospecimen research enterprises, within a single biorepository informatics system the vocabulary schema should be consistent.

Fortunately, there are a number of vocabulary standards from which terms can be drawn. SNOMED-CT and International Classification of Diseases (ICD) systems provide vocabularies and organizational ontologies for many clinical terms. ICD also includes organ topology codes that can be useful for defining anatomic sources of tissue biospecimens. The Foundational Model of Anatomy Ontology (FMA) is also an excellent source for anatomical site terms. The National Library of Medicine hosts the Unified Medical Language System (UMLS), which is a rich source of vocabularies for terms in both medicine and biology. The cancer protocols of the College of American Pathologists (CAP) provide a set of common data elements and vocabularies for tumor biospecimens. Perhaps the best sources for biospecimen-related vocabulary terms are the NCI's Cancer Data Standards Registry and Repository (caDSR) and Enterprise Vocabulary Services (EVS). This online "dictionary" and "thesaurus" of biomedical concepts, definitions, codes, and associated terms can provide a source of terms for biospecimen data systems, although they are biased for oncology-related terminologies and not specific for the domain of biospecimen science. A much more comprehensive terminology resource is hosted by the BioPortal website (http://bioportal.bioontology.org/), where virtually any medically related term may be concept coded using available ontologies.

User Interface

Although it is important that biospecimen data be represented consistently, accurately, and efficiently in any biorepository system, it is equally important that the user interface of any application be user friendly and designed to minimize time and effort for data entry tasks in the laboratory. Designing a user-friendly interface can be a particular challenge if data entry workflows differ among laboratories, protocols, or even specimen types that are using a common system. There are a number of traditional conventions or features within a user interface that can facilitate data entry for bank personnel and that should be a part of any well-designed system. These features include the use of barcode scanning for data entry; default data values that can be predefined at the patient, protocol, bank, or specimen levels; rational navigation between data fields within a data-entry screen using tab keys; an "auto-complete" feature in data fields that use a list of predefined data values; minimizing the number of "mouse clicks" or data screen changes required to enter data in a single data-entry session; and flexibility in navigating between different data-entry screens based upon changing workflows in the lab. Regardless of whether a system is being purchased or designed, it is essential that biobank staff end users play an active role in evaluating or specifying the functionality and features of the user interface because their extensive day-to-day, hands-on experience is valuable in determining which system interfaces would be most practical in the context of the laboratory environment. Without a properly designed interface, even the best-designed database could be severely lacking in the data intended to be collected if data entry tasks are too onerous or time consuming because of a poorly designed user interface.

Identifiers, Labeling, and Barcodes

Accurate, consistent, and unambiguous labeling of biospecimens and associated data objects is essential for the operation of a high-quality biorepository and/or biospecimen procurement service. For maintaining data integrity in a relational database schema, every data object (a patient, a biospecimen, a user, a freezer, a box, etc) is usually assigned a unique value, which is referred to as the *data table primary key.* This value is usually numeric, system generated, absolutely unique to the database, contains no intrinsic information, and is usually not used as a physical identifier for tracking biospecimens by the biorepository staff. Beyond this, a data object (such as a patient, a freezer, or a biospecimen) may be associated with additional identifiers. Some identifiers may be generated by external systems, such as surgical pathology case numbers or patient medical record numbers, and must be maintained in order to link biospecimens to data in other systems. Often such identifiers are not unique and are of varying format, although the combination of the identifier and the identifier source should confer uniqueness to the data object. For example, two tissue blocks received from a multi-institutional study may be labeled 09-1234 and a third block from the same study may be labeled SP09:1234. However, the combination of "09-1234" and "<ID_SOURCE='Christian NW Hospital'>" should confer uniqueness to the biospecimen. In another example, two patients participating in two different clinical studies may be identified by study number "12-002," but the combination of the study number together with the specific study in which the patient is enrolled should provide a unique identification of the patient and their corresponding biospecimens.

Beyond external identifiers and a database key, a biorepository may elect to assign an additional identifier to biospecimens, patients, storage containers, or other data objects. There are generally three approaches to assigning repository-specific identifiers. If a facility elects to use prelabeled tubes, plates, or adhesive labels for the physical storage and labeling of biospecimens, then an externally generated unique identifier (usually in the form of a barcoded alphanumeric string) may be assigned to the biospecimen. Generally, these data are then entered into the repository informatics system by scanning the physical barcode. This approach avoids potential errors in manual data entry and unintentional creation of duplicate identifiers; however, it does constrain the format and the method/workflow for which identifiers are assigned to objects in the data system. A converse approach is to allow the data system itself to generate unique identifiers and then physically assign those identifiers to biospecimens, containers, and other objects. A system-generated identifier can be guaranteed to be unique (at least within the system) and allows a flexible format design, including building intrinsic biospecimen information into the identifier itself (see below). Also, because the system can generate a new identifier at any time, it allows for the generation of a new identifier at any point in the data entry workflow. However, system-generated identifiers for biospecimens usually need to be printed to labels that can be physically attached to biospecimens and this may be inconvenient as compared to the use of prelabeled tubes or preprinted labels. A final approach employed by some systems is to allow a completely manual, ad hoc, user-defined identifier assignment (ie, the user types the desired identifier, usually chosen from a list or roster, in the data-entry screen). The system may or may not validate uniqueness of the assigned identifier; in either case, this approach should be avoided, if possible, because it can lead to numerous manual data-entry errors, incorrect identifier assignments, and potential creation of duplicate identifiers.

The format of the actual specimen identifier can vary. In cases where external identifiers are supplied from preprinted tubes or labels, the identifier is usually a long, user-*un*friendly, alphanumeric string that is also represented as a barcode. To guarantee uniqueness globally and over time, the identifier may be in the form of a Universally Unique Identifier (UUID) or use a similar convention that creates a label with an appearance similar to "147a9201-c23a-61b5-d346-113255760124." Data entry and query based on identifiers such as this can only be accurately and efficiently performed by barcode scanning and therefore imposes a hardware requirement that might not be available at all laboratory and/or clinical sites. In cases where the repository system itself is generating object identifiers, the format may be considerably more flexible. A popular approach is to include some intrinsic biophysical information about the specimen into the identifier itself. For example, all plasma samples collected in the laboratory might be labeled with a "P-" prefix, whereas all serum samples collected may be labeled with an "S-" prefix. In some approaches, specimens of different biophysical types collected from the same person or from the same person at the same point in time may use the same base identifier. For example, P-123 and S-123 would indicate a plasma and a serum sample, both collected from patient number 123. Similarly, some data systems may code provenance data within the identifier. For example, 123-PB1 may be assigned to a paraffin block collected from patient number 123. Then, 123-PB1-S3 might be the identifier of the third slide cut from paraffin block 1 from patient 123, and 123-PB1-S3-D1 might be the identifier of a DNA sample extracted from slide 3 cut from paraffin block 1 from patient 123. Although such labeling conventions can provide convenience for specimen identification by end users, they present many potential problems. As noted above, provenance-encoded identifiers can consist of long alphanumeric strings that may not easily fit on physical biospecimen labels. Such complex, alphanumeric identifiers can also be hard to sort or filter in data queries. Second, complex label-formatting rules may change over time and may not be applied consistently. For example, legacy serum samples collected before a specific date may not be labeled with an "S-" prefix, whereas those collected after that date may now contain the "S-" labeling convention. This situation can make searching and reporting on specimens on the basis of intrinsic specimen identifier information error-prone.

Another important problem occurs if information about the biophysical character or provenance of a biospecimen is entered incorrectly and subsequently corrected, because the specimen identifier itself will still probably contain incorrect information. For example, if a presumed serum specimen is collected from patient 123, assigned the identifier and physically labeled S-123, only to discover later that the specimen was a plasma specimen, this error can be corrected in the data system, but the biospecimen itself will still be labeled S-123 unless it is located, assigned a new identifier, and physically relabeled. For all of these reasons, it may be preferable to assign a unique numerical identifier to each specimen, but also provide additional human-readable information about the specimen on the physical specimen label, as desired. Thus, rather than a specimen identifier and physical label of S-123, an assigned biospecimen identifier (11267556) and physical label that appears as "11267556 / PT_ID: 123/Serum" will mitigate many of the biospecimen identification issues described above. Furthermore, with the appropriately designed software and hardware system, it should be possible to scan or enter unique specimen identifiers to rapidly retrieve all desired specimen data and more than could be possibly captured on a physical label.

Data Access

Functionality associated with data retrieval is a critical aspect of any intelligent biorepository informatics system. This includes both controlled access to data as well as actual searching and reporting features. If the data system is to be accessed by one or a few individuals who have identical roles with respect to the data, then a single-user, controlled-access (eg, password required) system sign-on may be sufficient. However, it is more likely, particularly for larger repositories, that multiple users with different roles may need access to the data. In these cases, role-based access is more appropriate, where each user is assigned specific permissions to add, edit, and view different types of data. Rationale for controlled data access may be regulatory, proprietary, and/or operational. Clinical staff and other appropriately credentialed personnel may be required to add, edit, and retrieve protected health information (PHI) data related to biospecimens and the patients from which they were collected. Such information may include names, dates, and medical record numbers. Repository staff and research scientists, however, may be restricted from viewing such PHI so that only de-identified or nonidentifying information can be viewed or updated. Depending upon the user's permissions, certain searches or data entry screens that contain PHI may be restricted. In cases where a repository and data system track specimens from multiple studies or trials, investigators may be concerned that their biospecimens, or even details of their study (such as study name), be visible and editable only to members within the study team and not to other researchers who may be searching for biospecimens collected under other studies or trials. Finally, if a repository system is designed to serve numerous facilities or storage sites simultaneously, it is important that staff within one physical repository location be restricted from editing or operating on specimen data related to specimens that are housed in a completely independent location.

The technical approaches for assigning data permissions to users are varied and outside of the scope of this chapter. However, when choosing or designing a biorepository data system, it is important to consider the current and potential future needs for restricting data to users on the basis of their functional role, association with a physical facility location, and involvement with specific protocols or collection activities.

Reporting

A well-designed biorepository informatics system should provide functionality for searching and reporting on biospecimen data. The scope of data searches (queries) and reports that are required will depend upon the users (investigators, administrators, biorepository staff and managers) who interact with the system. Simple systems may only provide predefined query capabilities that are not easily modified by end users. More sophisticated systems, however, may allow for the design, storage, and repeated execution of customized queries based on user-defined parameters. These parameters may include selection criteria for the query itself as well as the resulting data items that are to be displayed. It is important to carefully define and test queries to ensure that they return desired and expected results; therefore, customized queries should be constructed by individuals who are familiar both with biorepository inventory as well as query language.

Some systems may also allow query results themselves to be stored as biospecimen (or other data object) lists and allow results from multiple lists to be logically combined (*and, or, not*) to form new lists. Queries may involve identification of one or more specific biospecimens or biospecimen groups on the basis of user-defined parameters. Some searches may be straightforward: "Find all serum samples from African American women with a diagnosis of breast cancer"; but others may be more complex: "Find all patients with a diagnosis of breast cancer from whom both primary tumor tissue and a serum specimen, collected at least 6 months later, is available." The ability to form more complex queries will depend on appropriate representation of the data and on population of the system with complete and accurate data. As discussed previously, this requires intelligent design of the data model and simplified user interfaces that facilitate data entry.

Most query results are represented as simple lists of data items. These lists can often be exported to other analytical software packages such as SAS or Excel for additional formatting or analysis. For some repositories, it may be desirable to transfer individual biospecimen (object) level data directly to other external systems for billing or QA purposes (Figure 7-3). In addition, aggregate data may be transferred to systems such as the Common Biorepository Model (CBM), NCI Specimen Resource Locator, or other systems designed to advertise available biospecimen resources. However, it may also be useful for the biorepository data system itself to provide aggregate or cross-tabulated summary reports, particularly for common and repeated tasks. For example, monthly procurement reports, distribution/utilization reports, protocol or trial accrual statistics, and freezer inventories may be required as part of the biorepository QA process.

Security and Data Integrity

The security measures needed to protect biospecimen data systems will depend upon the data stored in the system as well as institutional information security practices. Systems that store only de-identified data and do not hold PHI will be less restricted. On first consideration, it may seem that an isolated desktop or local network system provides greater security because of its limited accessibility to external security threats; however, the eventual need to back up and transfer data on removable media or portable devices probably makes such a security approach more vulnerable to data piracy or unintentional data disclosure. In fact, industry-standard information technology can provide a secure environment for data storage and transfer through secure Internet protocols and is used routinely in the financial and health care industries. The design or purchase of any informatics system should include testing and validation of security measures, particularly through malicious Internet-based attacks if the system uses Internet-based data transfer. Several features of the software itself may facilitate good security practices, including user account management and provisioning for data access, as well as auditing (recording) and regular reporting of all data transactions (by user, date/time, and specific data transaction). It is important to note that although a software application may claim to be "21 CFR part 11 compliant" or "HIPAA compliant," conformation to such security standards is dependent upon not only the application itself, but also the policies and procedures under which it is used. Depending upon the local informatics environment, it may be possible to place the database (the physical data) behind a strong institutional security firewall while allowing an application server (the computer and software designed to collect and retrieve data to and from the database) to remain outside the firewall so that it can be accessed at remote sites. A "privileged" connection is then established between the application server and the database to provide highly regulated access to the physical data. Such exact hardware configurations will depend upon the policies of the institution's information security office.

In addition to preventing unauthorized access to data, it is important that a biorepository informatics system and the policies associated with its use protect the integrity of the data. The organization's information technology department (or the repository) should have clear policies for performing full and incremental data back-ups, off-site data storage, and restoration procedures.[3] Policies should also be in place for performing routine data audits, which may involve operational measures such as querying for 100 random biospecimens and validating their accurate location within the repository. It may also involve checks against external systems, such as validating the number and identity of participants enrolled in a particular protocol as compared to the same data that are represented in an associated CDMS. Sometimes executing queries with expected null results (eg, "Search for all prostate tissue specimens from female patients") can identify random or even systematic errors in data entry. Although data entry form controls utilized by the software (eg, use of restricted permissible value lists, required fields, and data-entry business logic) at the time of data entry should prevent such gross errors, frequent data auditing can identify unanticipated data-entry errors and permit rapid corrective action before significant compromise of the data occurs.

Hardware

Compared with other data sources encountered in biomedical research (eg, whole-slide image scans, massively parallel sequencing data, mass spectroscopy profiles, radiology images), biospecimen inventory and annotation data are relatively small. Hardware requirements for data storage, database operation, and application server functions (if relevant for the selected software solution) will depend upon the scope of biorepository operations and will mainly be related to the number of users and data transactions conducted per unit time. Configuration of the network within or outside of institutional security barriers (firewall) will be dictated by the user base that will access the system. All hardware systems should be equipped with appropriate data back-up mechanisms, physical security measures, and disaster-planning policies.[3] In all cases, it is important that the system (hardware and software) also be validated under "stress testing" conditions before being placed in a production environment, to ensure that system performance is maintained even beyond operations with the expected number of data records and simultaneous user data transactions. In particular, the time required for network-based data submissions and page loading in the production environment should be carefully documented, because impaired hardware or network performance during these operations (eg, a data-entry screen requiring 5 seconds versus 1 second to load) can severely affect usability and user acceptance of the system.

Perhaps even more important than the database and server hardware are components that are used within the biorepository for data entry. At a minimum, small form factor workstations or smart terminals should be located in key locations throughout the laboratory (eg, accessioning desk, processing bench, storage room) so as to allow easy and real-time access to the informatics system. Without immediate and direct accessibility in these locations, biospecimen data entry becomes post hoc, which can result in incomplete, delayed, or erroneous data being entered into the system. The use of touchscreen devices and barcode scanners (if supported by the software and laboratory workflow) can greatly expedite and encourage complete and accurate data entry. If secure wireless networking is available, tablet or other mobile devices that make use of cameras for barcode scanning may be used by the software application to accession biospecimens, log processing events, and record physical specimen transfers. This is particularly useful if a computer terminal with wired network access is not available in a location such as a clinical collection site, a processing bench, or a freezer inventory room.

References

1. Grizzle WE, Bell WC, Sexton KC. Issues in collecting, processing and storing human tissues and associated information to support biomedical research. *Cancer Biomark.* 2010;9(1-6):531-549.
2. Amin W, Singh H, Pople AK, et al. A decade of experience in the development and implementation of tissue banking informatics tools for intra and inter-institutional translational research. *J Pathol Inform.* 2010; Aug 10;1. pii:12.
3. Office of Biorepositories and Biospecimen Research, National Cancer Institute. *NCI Best Practices for Biospecimen Resources.* Washington, DC: National Institutes of Health, US Department of Health and Human Services; 2011. http://biospecimens.cancer.gov/practices/2011bp.asp. Accessed March 31, 2014.
4. Szirbik NB, Pelletier C, Chaussalet T. Six methodological steps to build medical data warehouses for research. *Int J Med Inform.* 2006; 75(9):683-691.
5. NCI Wiki. caTissue Suite. National Cancer Institute. https://wiki.nci.nih.gov/display/caTissue/caTissue+Suite. Accessed March 31, 2014.
6. Moore HM, Kelly A, Jewell SD, et al. Biospecimen reporting for improved study quality. *Biopreserv Biobank.* 2011;9(1):57-70.
7. Vaught JB, Henderson MK, Compton CC. Biospecimens and biorepositories: from afterthought to science. *Cancer Epidemiol Biomarkers Prev.* 2012;21(2):253-255.

Chapter 8

Biorepository Informed Consent Process

Nicole J. Sieffert

Informed Consent for Biospecimen Use in Research

The use of human biospecimens for research requires permission, with limited exception. Permission may come directly from the donor through the informed consent process or be granted by others charged with protecting the interests of the tissue donor. For the majority of biospecimen-related research, however, informed consent must be obtained from the specimen donor.

The concept of informed consent is founded on the principle of respect for autonomy and the notion that individuals have a right to control their medical care and research participation. This principle has both an ethical and a legal basis. This chapter presents a brief summary and overview of the processes and issues related to obtaining informed consent for the use of human specimens in research.

The Informed Consent Process

Informed consent is more than a form. It's a process. Its purpose is to protect the health and well-being of subjects by providing access to information required to make an informed decision regarding voluntary research participation. The process should also inform participants about their rights as research subjects. It begins when a potential subject is initially approached regarding research activity through face-to-face interaction, brochure receipt, video presentation, or review of a flyer, for example, and continues through study completion. Informed consent exists only when full disclosure of relevant information is presented to potential participants in a manner and language they understand. Potential participants should be able to choose freely and be competent to decide whether or not to participate in research.

Legally Effective Informed Consent

Informed consent is legally effective when it is obtained from the subject or the subject's legally authorized representative and is documented in a manner that is consistent with the US Department of Health and Human Services (HHS) protection of human subjects regulations and with applicable laws of the jurisdiction in which the research is conducted. It is important to note that the informed consent requirements in the regulations are not intended to preempt any applicable federal, state, or local laws that require additional information to be disclosed for consent to be legally effective (45 CFR 46.116(e)).[1]

The Common Rule

Federal regulations stipulate the general required elements of a valid informed consent document. These requirements apply equally to clinical treatment trials and research protocols without treatment aspects, including biobanking protocols. Requirements are codified in the Code of Federal Regulations (CFR) at 45 CFR 46.116 and 45 CFR 46.117,[2] referred to as the Common Rule, which governs human subjects research.

The HHS regulations, 45 CFR part 46, include four subparts: subpart A, also known as the *Federal Policy* or the *Common Rule;* subpart B, additional protections for pregnant women, human fetuses, and neonates; subpart C, additional protections for prisoners; and subpart D, additional protections for children. Each agency includes in its chapter of the CFR section numbers and language that are identical to those of the HHS codification at 45 CFR part 46, subpart A. The Common Rule outlines the basic provisions for Institutional Review Boards (IRBs), informed consent, and assurances of compliance for all participating departments and agencies. Human subject research conducted or supported by each federal department/agency is governed by the regulations of that department/agency. The head of that department/agency retains final judgment as to whether a particular activity it conducts or supports is covered by the Common Rule. Institutions seeking guidance on implementation of the Common Rule and other applicable federal regulations should contact the department/agency conducting or supporting the research.[3]

Exceptions to Application of the Common Rule

Research activities are exempt from the Common Rule if the only involvement of human subjects falls into one or more of the following categories.[4]

(1) Research conducted in established or commonly accepted educational settings, involving normal educational practices, such as (i) research on regular and special education instructional strategies, or (ii) research on the effectiveness of or the comparison among instructional techniques, curricula, or classroom management methods.

(2) Research involving the use of educational tests (cognitive, diagnostic, aptitude, achievement), survey procedures, interview procedures, or observation of public behavior, unless (i) information obtained is recorded in such a manner that human subjects can be identified, directly or through identifiers linked to the subjects; and (ii) any disclosure of the human subjects' responses outside the research could reasonably place the subjects at risk of criminal or civil liability or be damaging to the subjects' financial standing, employability, or reputation.

(3) Research involving the use of educational tests (cognitive, diagnostic, aptitude, achievement), survey procedures, interview procedures, or observation of public behavior that is not exempt under exception (2) above, if: (i) the human subjects are elected or appointed public officials or candidates for public office; or (ii) federal statute(s) require(s) without exception that the confidentiality of the personally identifiable information will be maintained throughout the research and thereafter.

(4) Research involving the collection or study of existing data, documents, records, pathologic specimens, or diagnostic specimens, if these sources are publicly available or if the information is recorded by the investigator in such a manner that subjects cannot be identified, directly or through identifiers linked to the subjects.

(5) Research and demonstration projects which are conducted by or subject to the approval of department or agency heads, and which are designed to study, evaluate, or otherwise examine: (i) public benefit or service programs; (ii) procedures for obtaining benefits or services under those programs; (iii) possible changes in or alternatives to those programs or procedures; or (iv) possible changes in methods or levels of payment for benefits or services under those programs.

(6) Taste and food quality evaluation and consumer acceptance studies, if: (i) wholesome foods without additives are consumed; or (ii) a food is consumed that contains a food ingredient at or below the level and for a use found to be safe, or agricultural chemical or environmental contaminant at or below the level found to be safe, by the Food and Drug Administration or approved by the Environmental Protection Agency or the Food Safety and Inspection Service of the US Department of Agriculture.

It is recommended, and often required, that determination of exemption be made and documented by the IRB, rather than assumed by an individual investigator.

Required Elements of Informed Consent

According to 45 CFR 46.116, obtaining "the legally effective informed consent of the subject or the subject's legally authorized representative" must be accomplished under circumstances "that provide the prospective subject... sufficient opportunity to consider whether or not to participate and to minimize the possibility of coercion or undue influence." Information provided to the prospective subject, whether in written or verbal form, must be in a language that the subject understands and may not contain "exculpatory language through which the subject or the representative is made to waive or appear to waive any of the subject's legal rights, or releases or appears to release the investigator, the sponsor, the institution, or its agents from liability for negligence."

The basic elements required to be provided to each subject when seeking to obtain informed consent include: (1) a statement that the study involves research, including its purposes, the expected duration of participation, descriptions of procedures to be followed, and identification of experimental procedures; (2) a description of reasonably foreseeable risks or discomforts; (3) a description of reasonably expected benefits, to the subject or to others; (4) a description of alternative procedures or treatments, if any; (5) a statement describing the extent to which confidentiality will be maintained; (6) for studies involving more than minimal risk, an explanation regarding whether any compensation for injuries are available and where to obtain further information; (7) information regarding whom to contact with questions about the research and research subjects' rights, and whom to contact regarding research-related injuries; and (8) a statement that participation is voluntary, refusal to participate won't involve any penalty or loss of benefits to which subjects are otherwise entitled, and that the subject may discontinue participation at any time without penalty or loss of benefits. See Table 8-1 for details regarding required elements of informed consent.

Table 8-1. Informed Consent Checklist: Basic Elements	
	A statement that the study involves research
	An explanation of the purposes of the research
	The expected duration of the subject's participation
	A description of the procedures to be followed
	Identification of any procedures which are experimental
	A description of any reasonably foreseeable risks or discomforts to the subject
	A description of any benefits to the subject or to others which may reasonably be expected from the research
	A disclosure of appropriate alternative procedures or courses of treatment, if any, that might be advantageous to the subject
	A statement describing the extent, if any, to which confidentiality of records identifying the subject will be maintained
	For research involving more than minimal risk, an explanation as to whether any compensation, and an explanation as to whether any medical treatments are available, if injury occurs and, if so, what they consist of, or where further information may be obtained
( ) Research Qs ( ) Rights Qs ( ) Injury Qs	An explanation of whom to contact for answers to pertinent questions about the research and research subjects' rights, and whom to contact in the event of a research-related injury to the subject
	A statement that participation is voluntary, refusal to participate will involve no penalty or loss of benefits to which the subject is otherwise entitled, and the subject may discontinue participation at any time without penalty or loss of benefits, to which the subject is otherwise entitled

Table 8-2. Informed Consent Checklist: Optional Elements	
1	A statement that the particular treatment or procedure may involve risks to the subject (or to the embryo or fetus, if the subject is or may become pregnant), which are currently unforeseeable
2	Anticipated circumstances under which the subject's participation may be terminated by the investigator without regard to the subject's consent
3	Any additional costs to the subject that may result from participation in the research
4	The consequences of a subject's decision to withdraw from the research and procedures for orderly termination of participation by the subject
5	A statement that significant new findings developed during the course of the research, which may relate to the subject's willingness to continue participation, will be provided to the subject
6	The approximate number of subjects involved in the study

Source: Office for Human Research Protections (http://www.hhs.gov/ohrp/policy/consentckls.html).

Optional Elements of Informed Consent

Additional informed consent elements may be preferred or required. Federal regulations stipulate six additional "optional" elements which may be required by the IRB, when appropriate (Table 8-2). These elements are not regulated by federal law but instead are based upon biobanking best practices and the recommendation of the authors.

The six federal requirements that may be required by an IRB include (1) a statement that a treatment or procedure may involve unforeseeable risks, (2) anticipated circumstances under which investigators may terminate subject participation without consent, (3) additional costs as result of participation, (4) procedures for and consequences of study withdrawal, (5) a statement that the subject will be provided with significant new findings developed during the study which may relate to his or her willingness to continue participation, and (6) the approximate number of subjects involved in the study. As readers may note, these six elements are routinely included in standard informed consent documents.

Maximizing the Clarity of Informed Consent: Additional Elements

Even when federal regulation requirements have been met, the inclusion of additional study-specific detail in the informed consent document may be essential to the decision-making process of the potential participant. Additional elements to be considered for inclusion in a biospecimen-related protocol are listed in Table 8-3. It is a best practice to include a response to each question and statement, providing as much information is deemed appropriate, in the informed consent document. The theme of these additionally recommended elements, as well as the required elements, is, as mentioned before, to provide prospective research participants with the information that a reasonable person would require to arrive at a decision about whether or not to participate in research.

Most states have legislation or legal cases that determine the required standard for informed consent. The three basic approaches include the following.[5]

- ***The reasonable physician standard:*** *What would a typical physician say about the interaction with the potential participant?* This standard allows the physician to determine what information is appropriate to disclose. It is probably not enough, however, since most research in this area shows that the typical physician tells the patient very little. This standard is also generally considered inconsistent with the goals of in-

Table 8-3. Additional Elements to be Considered for Inclusion in a Biospecimen-Related Protocol

General	Are Best Practices (NCI/BBRB, ISBER) being followed? Is the protocol related to a larger effort (collaborative groups, institutional banking efforts)?
People	Who manages biospecimens vs data? Who administers consent, handles revocation, and assures database-related updates regarding consent? Are all involved included in the study's Delegation of Authority Log?
Prospective Consent vs Waiver	List consent/waiver verification procedures. List waiver-specific details. Document the revocation response process.
Biospecimen Source	Are biospecimens prospectively collected, preexisting, or both? Are biospecimens obtained from clinical archives, as residual material from a clinical procedure, or collected exclusively for research? Are biospecimens collected only from the institution where the participant provided consent or from others as well (academic or other repositories, vendors, pharmaceutical companies)? If biospecimens will be obtained from other protocol collections within an institution, a protocol number should be provided. Has a provider agreement been obtained, if applicable? Desired biospecimen quantity should be stated (per individual, collection, and protocol). Risks involved in collection of the biospecimen quantity described above should be stated. Has the Division of Pathology or another department approved the intended biospecimen collection method?
Biospecimen, Derivative, and Data Sharing	State method of distribution and tracking biospecimens and data. If a Materials Transfer Agreement is established, provide details. List biospecimen and data recipient names, organizations, facilities. State distribution purpose (further research use vs testing/processing).
Biospecimen and Derivative Documentation and Tracking	List data elements to be collected and/or shared. State plans for data retention (form, length) and destruction (timing, method). Specify database use (type, access levels, security, standard operating procedures (SOP) for date entry updates).
Biospecimen Storage	State physical biospecimen storage location (resource, address, room, freezer, etc). Indicate temporary vs permanent storage. State intended storage term (length of time). State mechanisms of transfer, disposal, destruction. State guidelines for relocation upon: ▪ Principal investigator change or departure from institution or origin ▪ Protocol termination ▪ Repository closure (for any reason) State guidelines for disposal/destruction of unsuitable biospecimens.

formed consent, as the focus is on the physician rather than on what the patient needs to know.

- ***The reasonable patient standard:*** *What would the average patient need to know in order to be an informed participant in the decision?* This standard focuses on considering what a patient would need to know in order to understand the decision at hand.
- ***The subjective standard:*** *What would this potential participant need to know and understand in order to make an informed decision?* This standard is the most challenging to incorporate into practice, since it requires tailoring information to each potential participant.

Note that none of these implies an attempt to convey complete information, which may be impossible or undesirable. To borrow a bit of legal phraseology, we believe that the informed consent document should adhere to a "reasonable participant" standard. Perhaps the simplest way to conceptualize these elements is to envision the journey of the tissue specimen in question, from its origin with the participant through its procurement, handling, processing, use, storage, future use (if any), restocking, and ultimate depletion or disposal (see figure).[6]

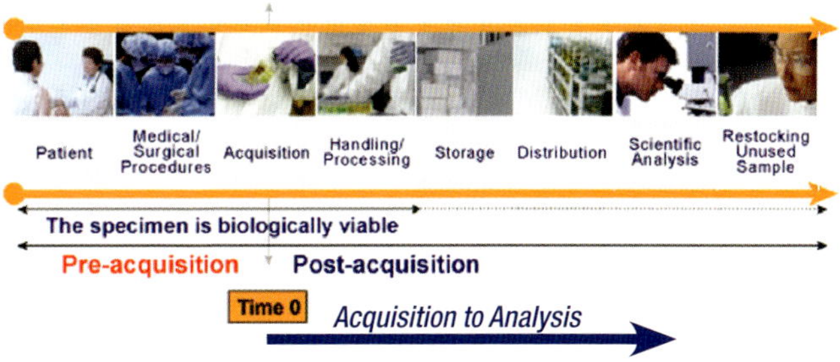

The goal should be to provide to the prospective participant a complete story of what will or may happen to samples provided. As with any good story, providing the who, what, when, where, why, and how is necessary and, in most cases, sufficient to inform the reasonable participant.

Table 8-3. Additional Elements to be Considered for Inclusion in a Biospecimen-Related Protocol (cont'd)	
Future Biospecimen Use	State intent or refusal to notify participant prior to biospecimen use.
Disclaimers	Biospecimen collection is dependent upon a variety of factors. Utilization is largely dependent upon QC standards. Patients should be told that consent does not guarantee collection, and that collection does not guarantee use. State that biospecimens collected for research are *not* intended for clinical use. The statement may be softened by adding, "We will make every effort to assist you, at our discretion, but are not obligated . . . ." In addition to biospecimen storage detail, state guidelines for biospecimen destruction upon study withdrawal. State whether or not participants may control/direct distribution or destruction of, directly withdraw, or otherwise influence biospecimen management.
Participant Options	Include available options regarding biospecimen use such as: ▪ Cell line creation ▪ Implantation in animals ▪ All research vs cancer research vs disease-specific research ▪ Genetic testing Include available options regarding future contact regarding: ▪ The initial study ▪ Future related studies ▪ Future unrelated studies ▪ Surveys ▪ Family member information *or* direct contact of family members
Biorepository-Specific Inclusions	Under what circumstances will biospecimens be used in the future? Avoid ". . . when approved by the IRB"-type statements. Describe the mechanism for determining authorization for future biospecimen use. Is release planned to other IRB-approved protocols within or outside of the institution of origin? Is application to the repository Director or Oversight Group required for biospecimen use? Define "leftover" (remnant/excess) as used at time of collection. Specify criteria for banking, primary distribution, secondary distribution, relocation/transfer (ownership unchanged), and destruction.

Abbreviations: NCI, National Cancer Institute; BBRB, Biorepositories and Biospecimen Research Branch; ISBER, International Society for Biological and Environmental Repositories; QC, quality control; IRB, Institutional Review Board.

Method of Consent

A consent document may be a full-form written document that embodies the elements of informed consent required by 45 CFR 46.116, or a short-form written consent document stating that the elements of informed consent required by 45 CFR 46.116 have been presented orally to the subject or the subject's legally authorized representative.

Paper Consent

The hard-copy consent document works well for consenting patients to provide tissue samples for research. This format is tried and true. It is the "gold standard." Patients, nurses, pathology staff, research administrators, and sponsors are accustomed to it. It is a tangible embodiment of what has been proposed to the prospective subject, indicating that he has agreed to those terms and is willing to participate under them. It may be read to the subject or the subject's legally authorized representative, but in any event, the investigator should give the subject or the representative adequate opportunity to read it before it is signed. The participant must be given a copy of the completed document, regardless of the consent format, and this effectively means a hard copy.

Utilization of paper consent documents has its shortcomings, however. One of the greatest is that papers may be lost. This is a continual problem for auditors and sometimes for investigators as well. Where verification of consent status becomes necessary prior to use or transfer of a sample, for instance, it may be necessary to physically locate each consent form to verify its legal sufficiency. Even for small protocols, in terms of number of participants, this is a daunting, laborious, resource-consuming task. When consent forms cannot be located, valuable samples and their associated data may have to be discarded according to the protocol, the IRB, institutional policy, and/or local regulations.

Paper consent documents, nevertheless, remain the standard format for obtaining informed consent for biospecimen-related research. We strongly encourage those administering paper consents for biobanking protocols to prospectively assure their legal adequacy and meticulously file and protect them, as biobanking studies may remain open and subject to audit and other duties for many years longer than the typical clinical research study.

Other methods of consent to be considered include electronic consent (document review and signature provided by the participant in the presence of a consent administrator), video consent (explanation of the informed consent by video followed by electronic participant signature), and web consent (web-based access to the informed consent document).

Electronic Consent

Electronic consenting is an emerging method of consent. It, too, has distinct advantages and disadvantages. Electronic consenting consists, at minimum, of participant consent documented in an electronic format. Electronic consent signature capture may include signing on a signature pad or capturing an electronic signature or a digital capture of the actual signature via touch screen. The signature capture system typically used is like one found at any of the myriad of electronic self-service kiosks encountered in everyday commercial life (for example, rental car counter or department store checkout).

Numerous commercial vendors of electronic consenting systems exist, and they are becoming increasingly common. Some have the ability to not only capture consent statute, but also to be used for information transmission, providing an electronic format for the verbatim text of the informed consent document as well as video and audio versions of the same, education materials, and links or access to other related information. In an increasingly electronic age, we favor the use of these devices when available, as they provide a means to convey a consistent and standardized message to prospective subjects and provide a means to easily maintain consent documents and consent status. The disadvantages of electronic consent include cost, training, and maintenance, any one of which can be beyond the reach of a typical study budget.

Video Consent

Video consenting should be explored. With this method, an IRB-approved script is used to create a video, which is then also IRB approved, to convey all of the elements of the consent document. The advantages of this method are that it is easily understandable and it presents the information to prospective participants in a manner in which they are accustomed to receiving information (ie, it's like watching TV). Unfortunately, however, the cost of production and the potential discomfort expressed by IRBs in relation to this method of consent may be a barrier. Another point of concern is that video may not be easily altered when revisions or changes are required. And let's not forget that the participant must be given a copy of the completed consent document. This means that a paper document will be generated and presented to the participant after the video is viewed and signature is obtained.

Web-Based Consent

Web-based consenting is an intriguing option. To our knowledge, it has not been successfully utilized to date as an initial consenting method for prospective biobanking research studies. It is an attractive notion, however, because it would allow prospective participants to consider participation at their leisure, at a place and time of their choosing. Individuals could investigate alternatives and take as much time as needed to reach a decision regarding participation. Hyperlinks could be provided to quickly respond to questions and to educate potential participants about virtually any aspect of the study.

The general public has grown increasingly comfortable with online transactions. A web-based consent system could allow participants to print their own copy of the signed consent document, assuming the technology existed to capture their signature at their workstation. The continuing difficulty with this method, however, is the difficulty in verifying the identity of the person consenting remotely. Indeed, another problem is verifying that the respondent is a human being and not a computer program designed to emulate provision of consent.

It is not clear to what extent or precisely how this problem should be solved before online consenting becomes a reality for biobanking protocols. We do, however, feel that it certainly should and can be solved. We find it interesting that financial transactions take place in the presence of precisely the same difficulties. It could be argued that the present risk to a person's well-being is of the same, if not a greater order of magnitude, in the midst of an electronic financial transaction than when providing permission to study remnant surgical tissue, yet millions of financial transaction occur online daily.

Timing of the Consent Process

The most appropriate time to approach a prospective subject for informed consent to provide biospecimens for research remains a matter of some debate. Most would agree that the informed consent process should take place an adequate distance in space and time from the actual procedure during which samples are obtained, given the federal requirement that informed consent be obtained in such a manner as to provide individuals with adequate opportunity to consider whether or not to participate, and that it remain free of coercion or undue influence.* The matter of debate is not the issue of approaching a surgical patient for consent to donate samples immediately preoperatively or after anesthesia has been administered, but instead, whether consent should be obtained before or after the tissue removal event.

We fall in the majority and believe that the proper time to administer consent for upcoming tissue removal procedures is before the procedure (and after the person has had an adequate opportunity to recover their mental capacity to make such a decision). For example, this model of consent timing requires that patients be consented preoperatively, before biopsies, and before phlebotomy. This removes any potential incentive for investigators to influence clinical care and engenders trust in both the clinical care and the research enterprise. It may mean the occasional lost opportunity, when desired tissue samples remain unavailable for research, but, as the old saying goes, it is better that a dozen murderers go free than to imprison an innocent man. And, in the end, some of these could be made available for research via other means (eg, obtaining a waiver of informed consent under an IRB-approved protocol to access clinical samples), so the opportunity is not always lost.

The general argument against consenting beforehand is that the prospective subject could be considered somewhat vulnerable and inherently susceptible to coercion or undue influence by their health care providers and the investigator, as they are effectually dependent upon them for their lives in some cases. The fear is that patients may not want to upset their health care providers by saying "no" to research. The extension of this line of logic concludes that people can make the most objective decision about whether or not to provide their tissue for research only after the physician–patient relationship has ended, which normally occurs at some time after the sample has been removed.

While intellectually persuasive, this "after" argument, we believe, has its own difficulties, and these difficulties make it a less optimal choice for timing of informed consent related to the provision of biospecimens. One difficulty is that, in most cases, the only materials that would be available under an after-the-fact consent are clinical materials. These clinical materials are subject to their own sets of rules and regulations requiring retention for stipulated periods of time and are required first and foremost for the clinical care of the person from whom they were ob-

* One could, we suppose, carry this rule of thumb too far and remove the consent process so far away in space–time as to be meaningless when it actually comes time to provide samples (think of consenting years in advance versus consenting days in advance).

tained. As such, they may be procured in a manner that makes them unsuitable for research purposes.** Additionally, it adds the logistical burden of having to find and re-contact patients at some time distant from their treatment.

Designing the Consent and Parental Permission Processes to Facilitate Understanding

Informed consent and parental permission language should be prepared in a way that is understandable and culturally sensitive to those being asked to participate or provide permission for participation of a minor. Subjects who do not speak English, for example, should be presented with a document written in a language that is understandable to them, and lay language should replace technical terms (eg, *blood draw* versus *venipuncture*). The Office for Human Research Protections (OHRP) strongly encourages the use of such a document whenever possible. (See OHRP guidance on this topic at http://www.hhs.gov/ohrp/policy/ic-non-e.html; for information about requirements for child assent, see FAQs regarding research with children.)

Limitations of Informed Consent

Although informed consent facilitates communication and decision making between physicians or their delegates and potential research participants, it does not, in itself, create an opportunity for autonomous choice. Consider, for example, a patient whose illness could be treated in many ways, but whose options are limited by a lack of medical insurance. The only real option for treatment may be one for which costs are paid through a research protocol. In this case, financial burdens limit the patient's freedom to freely choose whether or not to participate in that protocol.

Cultural issues may limit informed consent as well. Some non-Western cultures may not consider informed consent to be a universal ideal. In certain parts of the world, preserving community norms and family relationships is more important than the right of individuals to make decisions for themselves. In certain cultures, for example, women may be deemed incapable of making medical decisions for themselves; instead, that right is given to husbands or fathers. In other cases, patients may prefer to avoid bad news or to delegate decision-making responsibilities to family members. In practice, negotiating the balance between respect for autonomy and a patient's desire for information or decision-making authority can be difficult.[7]

Consent Document Format

Because the goal of any informed consent process is to adequately inform prospective subjects, format does matter. An explanation of what will happen to donated tissue samples must be presented in an understandable manner, as illustrated by the federal requirements to have the information provided in an understandable language, without coercion or undue influence, and as illustrated in the frequently required element of relatively low reading levels for comprehension of consent documents.

In our experience, part of the ability to meaningfully convey the story of donated tissue depends upon where the required and optional elements are found in the informed consent document. The consent elements must be grouped in a way that makes sense in order for the potential participant to understand what is planned for donated samples and what it means to provide those samples. Scattering elements throughout an informed consent document makes it difficult, even for experienced readers, to locate specific tissue-related elements and to understand the life cycle of donated samples. A dictionary is a fitting analogy; it certainly contains the words necessary to write a book, but they are out of context. In the same way, presentation of consent elements out of context relative to one another fails to adequately convey the detailed plan to which the potential participant is asked to consent. We therefore recommend the adoption, as a standard process, of providing in informed consent documents, at minimum, a single section designated for the simple, concise description of consent elements and relevant details related to the biospecimen life cycle including, but not limited to, tissue procurement, processing, storage, future use, distribution, and disposal.

Models of Consent for Biorepositories

Informed consent documents may be structured in a variety of ways to accommodate a particular process or research goal. Models of consent for biorepository use include the following.

Presumed Consent ("Opting Out")

Presumed consent stands in stark contrast to conventional methods of seeking informed consent. In

** For example, most clinical samples do not require snap-freezing upon collection, while many research studies require snap-freezing of procured samples.

this "opt out" system, consent is presumed, and individuals are required to document the wish to be uninvolved in research. A number of arguments exist against the use of this model, including the danger of using patients as a means to an end, as autonomy is overridden without consent to a specific action.

Broad Consent

In general, broad consent is intended to allow the use of biospecimens and related data in immediate and future research of any kind at any time. This model is frequently used by biorepositories and is favored because it allows the repository or its governing body to determine how best to utilize its collections. This format includes all of the required elements and often additional optional elements as well. It combines the potential benefit of additional research with a low level of risk when adequate measures are in place to protect privacy and confidentiality. It has been argued, however, that the absence of specific information regarding future specimen use prohibits autonomy, rendering the consent process unethical. We believe that broad consent is ethical in that it asks potential participants to consent to allow governance of donated specimens, and that asking the individual to choose whether or not to participate is a display of respect for autonomy, which is itself the primary justification of the requirement to obtain informed consent.[8]

Broad consent should include a general description of the biorepository as an indication of the type of research generally conducted, an explanation as to how specimen use decisions will be made, some reference to the goals of the research to be conducted using repository resources, and a description of the controlling institution's mission and values.

Partially Restricted Consent

The partially restricted model of informed consent allows the use of biological specimens and related data in specific immediate research and in future investigations directly or indirectly associated with them. Restrictions may be related to types of specimens to be collected and used, types of research to be performed, and limits placed upon future use, among other things. A partially restricted form of consent for biorepositories balances the sometimes conflicting interests of donor autonomy and medical research by informing the sample donor about the parameters of potential specimen use. This format may be utilized as an institutional "front door" consent, for example, when specimens collected are residual (post patient care) and risk is minimal.

Multilayered Consent

Multilayered consent requires several options to be explained to the potential research participant using a detailed form. This type of consent document may be paired with an information letter, directed to potential participants, containing specific information about the storage of biological samples and related data; the nature and purposes of the studies to be carried out; general information about studies that could be developed in the future in association with the original research; specific information regarding privacy; donor authorization for use of anonymous samples and data for scientific publications, teaching purposes, or commercialization; specific information on the right of the donors to request and obtain details of the status of the work and general study results; and specific information about the right to withdraw consent and request the destruction or irreversible anonymization of samples and data.

The layered consent form itself may include the donor's consent to store samples and related data; consent to specific studies and associated future investigations; consent to use results from these studies for scientific publications, teaching purposes, or commercial products; and the donor's declaration that he has been informed of the right to withdraw consent at any time and that he has been informed of the right to request the results obtained from use of the biological samples and related data, although inclusion of this point requires thoughtful consideration.

Specific (Fully Restricted) Informed Consent

Specific informed consent (also referred to as fully-restricted or protocol-specific consent) allows the use of biological specimens and related data only in immediate research and forbids any future study that is not foreseen at the time of the original consent. This format is particularly useful for studies in which biospecimen use is targeted, as in the case of disease-specific studies.

Documentation of Informed Consent

Informed consent is most often documented in written form to include key information regarding the research in which a participant is involved. The consent form is intended, in part, to provide information for the subject's reference and to document the interaction between the subject and the investigator or his representative. The completed consent document alone, however, does not constitute completion of the consent process. Potential participants must be given an opportunity to consider the consent document details and to ask questions—and even this must be documented.

Obtaining and Documenting Consent for Non–English-Speaking Participants

The HHS regulations for the protection of human subjects require that informed consent information be presented "in language understandable to the subject" and, in most situations, that informed consent be documented in writing (45 CFR 46.116 and 46.117). The written consent document should include all the elements required for legally effective informed consent.

The CFR does, however, permit oral presentation of informed consent information in conjunction with a short-form written consent document (stating that the elements of consent have been presented orally) and a written summary of what is presented orally. A witness to the oral presentation is required, and the subject must be given copies of the short-form document and the summary.[9] The oral presentation and the short-form document must be in a language that is understandable to the potential participant, and the witness should be fluent in English as well as the potential participant's language. It is the responsibility of the IRB to determine which method is appropriate for documenting informed consent obtained from non–English-speaking participants and to approve all short forms when their use is deemed appropriate.

Consent With Diminished Decision-Making Capacity

The HHS regulations are silent on consent procedures specific to subjects with impaired decision-making capacity, as in the case of mental retardation, some forms of mental illness, or dementia, or as the result of trauma, whether temporary, progressive, or permanent. The regulations do require that the IRB ensure that "additional safeguards have been included in the study to protect the rights and welfare" of all subjects that are "likely to be vulnerable to coercion or undue influence." The regulations include "mentally disabled persons" in this category (45 CFR 46.111(b)).

In studies involving progressive disorders or aging populations, participants may initially be competent to consent on their own behalf but may experience effects of progressive or intermittent disorders that lead to decisional impairment during the course of the study. In cases such as this, it is appropriate to discuss the possibility of a legally authorized representative with the prospective participants.

Consent in an Urgent Setting

Because individuals receiving urgent or emergent medical care may be vulnerable to coercion or undue influence—even if temporarily—additional protections may be required to ensure the subject's consent to participate in research is truly voluntary and is sought under circumstances that minimize the possibility of coercion or undue influence (45 CFR 46.111(b), 45 CFR 46.116). In some cases, it might be possible to obtain consent from a legally authorized representative (eg, in the case of incapacitated individuals). In certain emergency circumstances, the Secretarial waiver of informed consent under 45 CFR 46.101(i) may be applicable. It should be noted that if the research is regulated by FDA, the Secretarial waiver permits the research to be conducted under a comparable provision.[10]

Minimizing the Possibility of Coercion or Undue Influence

The HHS regulations state that "an investigator shall seek such consent only under circumstances that provide the prospective subject or the representative sufficient opportunity to consider whether or not to participate and that minimize the possibility of coercion or undue influence" (45 CFR 46.116). This requirement applies to all nonexempt human subjects research not eligible for a waiver of the consent requirements.[1]

Coercion occurs when an overt or implicit threat of harm is intentionally presented by one person to another in order to obtain compliance.[11] An investigator might imply that a prospective subject will lose access to needed health services, for example, if he does not participate in research.[1]

Undue influence, by contrast, often occurs through an offer of an excessive or inappropriate reward or other overture in order to obtain compliance.[11] An investigator might, for example, promise students extra credit for research participation; undue influence is present if no alternate means of extra credit exists. The same is true, although in more subtle form, when patients are approached for research participation by caregivers who are also investigators. The patient may feel obligated to participate in the caregiver's studies.[1]

Because of the relative nature and lack of clear-cut standards on the boundaries of inappropriate and appropriate forms of influence, investigators and IRBs must be vigilant about minimizing the possibility of coercion and undue influence. Reasonable accommodations can be made to minimize the likelihood of undue influence or coercion. Known participant benefits should be stated accurately, but not exaggerated, and potential or uncertain benefits should be noted as such, with clear language indicating how much is known about the uncertainty or likelihood of these potential benefits.[1]

Regulatory requirements for IRB review and approval also specify the need for the IRB, in order to approve research covered by the HHS regulations, to ensure that "when some or all of the subjects are likely to be vulnerable to coercion or undue influence, such as children, prisoners, pregnant women, mentally disabled persons, or economically or educationally disadvantaged persons, additional safeguards have been included in the study to protect the rights and welfare of these subjects" (45 CFR 46.111(b)). Thus, inducements that would ordinarily be acceptable in some populations may become undue influences for these vulnerable subject groups.[1]

Requirements for Assent and Parental Permission in Research With Children

By regulatory definition, children are "persons who have not attained the legal age for consent to treatments or procedures involved in the research, under the applicable law of the jurisdiction in which the research will be conducted" (45 CFR 46.402(a)). In the United States, the legal age of adulthood is a matter of state and local law. This means that adulthood may vary from state to state. In a large majority of states, 18 years is the legal age of adulthood, but this is not true in every state, locality, or territory. State law may also address circumstances in which a person below the age of adulthood is legally authorized to consent to medical procedures, as with contraceptives. Certain states provide a mechanism for the emancipation of minors, through which a child younger than the legal age of adulthood may gain certain civil rights, which might include the legal ability to consent to research participation.

The definition of children also takes into account the particular interventions or interactions involved in the proposed research (eg, surveys, blood tests). For example, in some places, individuals who are 16 years of age may legally consent to certain clinical interventions or interactions. If the involvement of human subjects in a proposed research activity consists of these interventions or interactions, then those individuals may be considered as adults for that purpose. If a proposed activity includes an intervention or interaction for which the subject has not yet reached the legal age of consent, however, that person must be considered a child.[1]

Assent is a child's affirmative agreement to participate in research. The IRB is responsible for deciding whether child assent is required in proposed research activities. Mere failure to object should not, absent affirmative agreement, be construed as assent (45 CFR 46.402(b)).

Child assent is required, except in the following three circumstances described at 45 CFR 46.408(a): (1) the capability of some or all of the children is so limited that they cannot reasonably be consulted; (2) the intervention or procedure involved in the research holds out the prospect of direct benefit to the health or well-being of the children and is available only in the context of the research; and (3) the research meets the same conditions as those for waiver or alteration of informed consent in research involving adults, as specified in the regulations at either 45 CFR 46.116(c) or 45 CFR 46.116(d).

The IRB must determine, to the extent required by 45 CFR 46.116, that adequate provisions are made for soliciting the assent of the children, when in the judgment of the IRB, the children are capable of providing assent, as well as the permission of the parents (45 CFR 46.408). Permission means the agreement of one or both parents or a guardian to the participation of a child or ward in research (45 CFR 46.402(c)). Under 45 CFR 408(b), the IRB may find that the permission of one parent is sufficient for research to be conducted under 45 CFR 46.404 or 45 CFR 46.405. Where research is conducted under 45 CFR 46.406 or 45 CFR 46.407, permission must be obtained from both parents unless one parent is deceased, unknown, incompetent, or not reasonably available, or when only one parent has legal responsibility for the care and custody of the child.

If the IRB determines that the capability of some or all of the children is so limited that they cannot reasonably be consulted regarding assent, or that the intervention or procedure involved in the research holds out a prospect of direct benefit that is important to the health or well-being of the children and is available only in the context of the research, the assent of the children is not a necessary condition for proceeding with the research. Even when the IRB determines that the subjects are capable of assenting, the IRB may still waive the assent requirement under certain circumstances in accord with 45 CFR 46.116 and 45 CFR 46.408(a).

Table 8-4. Documentation of Informed Consent	
Written	The consent form may be either of the following: 1. A **written consent** document that embodies the elements of informed consent required by §46.116. This form may be read to the subject or the subject's legally authorized representative, but in any event, the investigator should give either the subject or the representative adequate opportunity to read it before it is signed.
Done Orally	2. A **short form written consent** document, stating that the elements of informed consent required by §46.116 have been presented **orally** to the subject or the subject's legally authorized representative. When this method is used, there shall be a **witness** to the oral presentation. Also, the IRB shall approve a **written summary** of what is to be said to the subject or the representative. Only the short form itself is to be signed by the subject or the representative. However, the witness shall sign both the short form and a copy of the summary, and the person actually obtaining consent shall sign a copy of the summary. A copy of the summary shall be given to the subject or the representative, in addition to a copy of the short form.
Waiver of Requirement for Signed Form	An IRB may waive the requirement for the investigator to obtain a signed consent form for some or all subjects, if it finds either: 1. That the only record linking the subject and the research would be the consent document, and the **principal risk** would be potential harm resulting from a breach of confidentiality. Each subject will be asked whether the subject wants documentation linking the subject with the research, and the subject's wishes will govern; or 2. That the research presents **no more than minimal risk** of harm to subjects, and involves no procedures, for which written consent is normally required outside of the research context. In cases in which the documentation requirement is waived, the IRB may require the investigator to provide subjects with a written statement regarding the research.

Abbreviation: IRB, Institutional Review Board.
Source: Office for Human Research Protections (http://www.hhs.gov/ohrp/policy/consentckls.html).

Supplementing Initial Consent or Parental Permission

Ensuring an adequate consent or parental permission process may require repeating or supplementing the initial consent procedure. The HHS regulations stipulate that "an investigator shall seek such consent only under circumstances that provide the prospective subject or the representative sufficient opportunity to consider whether or not to participate and that minimizes the possibility of coercion or undue influence" (45 CFR 46.116). This requirement may also necessitate repeating or supplementing the initial consent procedure. Informed consent and parental permission should be viewed as an ongoing process.

Documenting Child Assent

The IRB has the discretion to determine the appropriate manner, if any, of documenting child assent. The IRB should decide what form of documentation, if any, is most appropriate, based on such considerations as the child's age, maturity, and degree of literacy. The HHS regulations do not require documentation of assent. If adolescents are involved in research where a consent form would have been used if the subjects were adults, it would generally be appropriate to use a similar form to document an adolescent's assent.[6]

If young children are involved who are unable to read, documentation should take a form that is appropriate for the purpose of recording that assent took place. The IRB may also decide that documentation of assent is not warranted. See the Table 8-4 for details regarding required documentation of informed consent.

The consent process and its documentation should be revised when deficiencies in its accuracy or completeness are noted, when new information about reasonably foreseeable risks and potential benefits becomes available, or when other additional information becomes known that will improve the consent process. Such revisions must be reviewed and approved by the IRB prior to the revised consent being utilized except when necessary to eliminate apparent immediate hazards to subjects (45 CFR 46.103(b)(4)).

Waiving or Altering the Requirement for Documentation of Informed Consent or Parental Permission

Parental or guardian permission for research involving children can be waived under certain circumstances. An IRB may waive the requirements for obtaining parental or guardian permission if either of the following two conditions is met: (1) the IRB finds and documents that the research is to be conducted by or subject to the approval of state or local government officials and is designed to study, evaluate, or otherwise examine (a) public benefit or service programs, (b) procedures for obtaining benefits or services under those programs, (c) possible changes in or alternatives to those programs or procedures, or (d) possible changes in methods or levels of payment for benefits or services under those programs (45 CFR 46.116(c)(1)); and (2) the research could not practicably be carried out without the waiver or alteration (45 CFR 46.116 (c)(2)).

The IRB may also waive the requirements for obtaining parental or guardian permission if it determines that a research protocol is designed to study conditions in children or a subject population for which parental or guardian permission is not a reasonable requirement to protect the subjects, as in the case of neglected or abused children, and the following two additional criteria are also met: (1) an appropriate mechanism is in place to protect the children; and (2) the waiver is not inconsistent with federal, state, or local law (45 CFR 46.408(c)).

The choice of an appropriate substitute mechanism (for example, appointing a child advocate or an assent monitor) for protecting children participating in research would depend on the nature and purpose of the activities described in the protocol, the risk and anticipated benefit to the research subjects, and the child's age, maturity, status, and condition (45 CFR 46.408(c)). Note that an IRB may waive the requirement for obtaining parental or guardian permission under 45 CFR 46.408(c) even if the research involves more than minimal risk to the child subjects.

General Recommendations

We endorse the following "best practices" when developing, administering, and documenting the informed consent process:

- Acknowledgement of varied education and literacy levels among potential participants, and provision of additional assistance for those who are less educated or less literate
- Language use at lower reading levels (ie, eighth grade); consistent formatting to include required, optional, and best-practice elements; graphics, when appropriate; and concise content overall
- Use of a standard basic template for the creation of informed consent documents to ensure appropriate content and consistent language
- Use of consent forms as an outline for discussion with potential participants to ensure the presentation of key information
- Use of multimedia formats (eg, webcasts, DVDs), whenever possible, and written information to improve understanding
- Allowance of time for extended discussion with potential participants to permit an opportunity for open discussion and consideration of participation without undue pressure
- Use of the "teach back" method in which patients are asked to repeat the information that has been presented to them
- Distribution of quick reference/summary/fact sheets to participants for later reference

It is the role of the consent administrator to ensure that potential participants understand the voluntary nature of research participation, feel comfortable taking the time required to evaluate the request to participate, and are confident that all questions and concerns have been appropriately addressed. As mentioned earlier, informed consent is a process that must be handled appropriately to be deemed valid.

Conclusions

Active protection of patients' interests in the research participation decision-making process is an indication of respect for individual integrity. It requires respectful dialogue with patients about their circumstances and care. Sensitivity to the limitations of and tensions inherent in patient-centered medical decision making is absolutely necessary. Truly informed decision making is compromised when institutional structures and processes fail to provide adequate opportunities for physician–patient communication.[7] Legal and regulatory guidance alone, though essential, is not enough to ensure truly informed consent. Thoughtful consideration of the informed consent process and its carefully constructed implementation and oversight are indispensible components of ethically conducted research.

References

1. US Department of Health and Human Services. Informed Consent - FAQs. http://answers.hhs.gov/ohrp/categories/1566. Accessed March 31, 2014.
2. US Department of Health and Human Services. General requirements for informed consent. CFR 46 § 46.116. http://www.hhs.gov/ohrp/humansubjects/guidance/45cfr46.html#46.116. Revised January 15, 2009. Effective July 14, 2009. Accessed March 31, 2014.
3. US Department of Health and Human Services. Federal Policy for the Protection of Human Subjects ('Common Rule'). http://www.hhs.gov/ohrp/humansubjects/commonrule/index.html. Accessed March 31, 2014.
4. US Department of Health and Human Services. To what does this policy apply?. CFR 46 § 46.101. http://www.hhs.gov/ohrp/humansubjects/guidance/45cfr46.html. Revised January 15, 2009. Effective July 14, 2009. Accessed March 31, 2014.
5. University of Washington School of Medicine. Ethics in Medicine. Informed consent. http://depts.washington.edu/bioethx/topics/consent.html. Accessed March 31, 2014.
6. Biorepositories and Biospecimen Research Branch, National Cancer Institute. *Lifecycle of Biospecimens.* http://biospecimens.cancer.gov/researchnetwork/lifecycle.asp. Accessed October 2, 2013.
7. del Carmen G, Joffe S. Informed consent for medical treatment and research: a review. *Oncologist.* 2005; 10(8):636-641. http://theoncologist.alphamedpress.org/content/10/8/636.full. Accessed March 31, 2014.
8. Beauchamp T, Childress J. *The Principles of Biomedical Ethics.* 6th ed. Oxford, UK: Oxford University Press; 2008.
9. Lin MH; Office for Human Research Protections (OHRP). Memorandum, November 9, 1995. http://www.hhs.gov/ohrp/policy/ic-non-e.html. Accessed March 31, 2014.
10. Office for Human Research Protections. Informed consent requirements in emergency research. *OPRR Reports.* October 31, 1996. http://www.hhs.gov/ohrp/policy/hsdc97-01.html. Accessed March 31, 2014.
11. National Commission for the Protection of Human Subjects of Biomedical and Behavioral Research. *The Belmont Report. Ethical Principles and Guidelines for the Protection of Human Subjects of Research.* Washington, DC: National Institutes of Health, Department of Health, Education, and Welfare, Office of Human Subjects Research; April 18, 1979. http://www.hhs.gov/ohrp/humansubjects/guidance/belmont.html. Accessed March 31, 2014.

Chapter 9

Cost Assessment for Developing an Institutional Biorepository

Scott Jewell
Dana Valley
Dan Rohrer

It is virtually impossible to provide a clear, clean process to determine the costs of developing a biorepository. Simply stated, it is an exercise in discovery of what is needed and the amount of support that will become available. Planning, which is critical for the development of a biorepository, is best accomplished with a clear assessment of the purpose and goals of the biorepository. Stakeholders need to be included in the development, as well as users consulted and management structures considered. In addition, specialists in informatics systems must be involved to help determine what level of sophistication is needed in information technology. Especially important is the connectivity to clinical data that is associated with the biospecimens, while maintaining systems of participant confidentiality. An institutional resource like a biorepository will need to function within the jurisdiction of several other institutional departments, such as the Institutional Review Board (IRB), Privacy Office (if different from the IRB), the Compliance Office for Laboratory Safety, Human Resources, Facilities, and Administration. All of these departments should be made aware of the purposes and functions of the biorepository and ensure that the planning is complete in order to best assess the overall start-up costs and annual operating costs.

Mission-Related Cost and Biorepository Value

Large biorepositories holding millions of biospecimens can cost millions of dollars to develop and operate. Examples of some sites for such biorepositories include the Centers for Disease Control and Prevention[1]; the National Heart, Lung, and Blood Institute[2]; the Department of Defense Joint Pathology Center[3]; and the Coriell Institute for Medical Research.[4] Several institutes of the National Institutes of Health maintain a biorepository to support research. In addition, many pharmaceutical companies manage very large biorepositories. Several of these and other mega-biorepositories are funded by the federal government or large industry applications, which may suggest that a single academic institution cannot meet the same standards that are placed on the mega-biorepositories; however, the elements of best practices and general infrastructure are similar and often applicable from the largest to the smallest of biorepositories. An academic research biorepository is most often established at the institution's hospitals, colleges, or departments for a group of researchers and then eventually becomes a central infrastructure resource.

Biorepositories are generally supported by a combination of grant and department funding, but because biorepositories are considered, mistakenly, to be a simple infrastructure and able to be manageable by anyone, often very little planning goes into developing these central resources appropriately. Furthermore, central biorepositories may be avoided because of the perception that trained staff are not needed, that staff employed specifically for a biorepository cost too much, and that the biorepository should be managed by individual investigators. It is interesting to note that if an investigator purchases a freezer and stores laboratory-generated materials (cell lines, reagents, or products), there is no expectation that this resource should generate any income. The materials are not accessible to anyone else and distribution guidelines are more easily breached, which would create a level of risk for the institution. On the other hand, central biorepositories are expected to generate payback charges or revenue, and whereas investigators' grants help pay for their personally collected biospecimens, a central biorepository does not receive grants. Viewing the biorepository in this light—as an overburdening cost—does not take into account the complete picture. Consideration for a central biorepository should be based first on the value to the institution. If planned accordingly, a centrally managed biorepository can manage institutional costs and risks because it will accomplish the following:

- Provide an organized system for the collection, processing, and storage for easier access to biospecimens by investigators, reducing the time and effort for the investigators' staff.

- Reduce the footprint of freezers, thereby saving space and institutional electrical and HVAC costs.
- Provide an organized security for the appropriate access to freezers and biospecimens.
- Provide organized protocols to ensure high-quality biospecimens and proper management of these specimens.
- Ensure proper service maintenance to prevent freezer failures.
- Provide organized backup emergency options to protect the critical investments of the research.

The value of biorepositories to institutions has been witnessed by examples of courtroom decisions where the issue of ownership of biospecimens has been debated.[5-7] The College of American Pathologists has developed a Biorepository Accreditation Program[8] to help improve the overall quality of the operations of biorepositories. Furthermore, with increasing regulatory concerns regarding the identifiability of DNA in biospecimens or that research results should be made available to subjects, a properly managed central biorepository may be the best management of biospecimens that institutions can introduce to minimize the risk in human subjects research.[9,10]

When centrally managed biorepositories are developed as a resource for researchers to collect tissues from surgery or to support banked clinical trial biospecimens, the investment can be helpful and rewarding. Unfortunately, biorepository resources will not be able to reimburse the institution for their total costs of operation. However, if managed well, the assessment of the costs can be counted as a positive investment toward generating research funding through individual investigator grants, program project grants, Specialized Programs of Research Excellence (SPORE) grants, and specialized applications.

Assessment of the Biorepository Translates to Cost

The International Society for Biological and Environmental Repositories (ISBER) has published two tools—*2012 Best Practices for Repositories*[11] and a Self-Assessment Tool (SAT)[12]—for its membership that assist in the evaluation of repositories, both in function and cost. The Best Practices document provides the framework for what can be considered necessary in a biorepository, which depends on the scope of the particular biorepository. Examples of the headings in the Best Practices document are listed in Table 9-1. A very similar set of topics can also be found published by the Biorepositories and Biospecimen Research Branch (BBRB) at the National Cancer Institute (NCI).[13] Using either the ISBER or NCI Best Practices followed by the ISBER SAT, an institution can begin to evaluate where they are relative to the costs required for developing a biorepository. In some situations, institutions may already have some existing resources that can be leveraged for the infrastructure, such as equipment, space, or resources. Once these existing resources have been evaluated and new resources required have been identified, a budget for start-up and also for annual costs can be produced.

Biorepository Budgets: Revenue Minus Expenses Equals Subsidy

A detailed sample spreadsheet for a biorepository with multiple, well-funded projects and subprojects is shown in Table 9-2. Each line item under "DESCRIPTION" would have an associated spreadsheet as seen in Table 9-3, with the details of the costs for those areas. The detail may help a beginning biorepository select relevant section of interest. The spreadsheet also provides an example of the scope of items that may be needed in a biorepository. The budget includes revenue from grants as well as institutional funds or support. Each expense and revenue of a central biorepository should be tracked for as many projects as possible. It is also important to verify that the project goals have been met. The example shown in Table 9-3 is not an exhaustive list of elements to be tracked because no two biorepositories are exactly alike. The example is based on a real biorepository system, and, in the end, the assessment is measured as an institutional investment of $1.1 million dollars of a $4.1 million dollar operating budget. The institution's investment is 26.8% of the total budget, and this does not include indirect costs that are captured by the institution. As noted, biorepositories are most often not a zero sum operation, which is not to indicate that a well-designed and managed biorepository can't get close to a break-even operation, but it is not the norm. A biorepository is an institutional resource investment, much like the information technology network and other resources of the institution.

Regarding the reimbursements, or chargeback fees, for the use of biospecimens, institutions generally determine the fees based on the overall costs of operation. For-profit companies charge fees that must maintain a profit opportunity, and therefore their fees will be much higher than those of an individual academic institution. Biospecimens with small or un-

Table 9-1. Categories of Best Practices and Areas of Assessment

Personnel	Manager	Standard operating procedures Informed consent Institutional Review Board documentation
	Laboratory technologist	
Information Technology	Office software	
	Bioinventory software	
	Barcode readers/technology	
Equipment	Freezers	
	Freezer inventory	
	Computers	
	Office equipment	Desks, chairs, document cabinets, phones, fax, copiers
Space	Office	
	Repository	
	Laboratory	
	Location – proximity	
Products	Specimen processing materials	
	Office materials	Informed consent Brochures for patients Application documents Biospecimen agreements
	Time and effort	Informatics personnel Technologist personnel Managerial personnel Informed consent process

Table 9-2. Example of an Annual Budget Sheet for a Biorepository

RESEARCH INSTITUTE
BUDGET FY 2014
TOTAL BUDGET SUMMARY

	Project A				Project B				Project C			
DESCRIPTION	Biobank 1	Biobank 2	Biobank 3	Biobank 4	Biobank 1	Biobank 2	Biobank 3	Biobank 4	Biobank 1	Total Grants	Total Internal	Total
Direct External Revenue	$ 509,444	$ 754,563	$ 861,471	$ 442,779	$ 5,000	$ 400,000	$ -	$ -	$ -	$ 2,568,257	$ 405,000	**$2,973,257**
Capital Equipment	66,500	-	-	-	-	-	-	-	-	66,500	-	**66,500**
Salaries & Wages	243,875	321,485	335,341	144,943	179,905	370,267	15,089	67,678	103,227	1,045,644	736,165	**1,781,810**
Other Compensation	-	-	89,173	-	7,500	1,100	-	-	-	89,173	8,600	**97,773**
Benefits	68,285	90,016	93,895	40,584	38,475	86,324	3,518	15,746	24,066	292,780	168,130	**460,910**
Equipment / Software	-	-	-	-	14,500	7,000	500	1,000	-	-	23,000	**23,000**
Lab Supplies & Services	99,051	52,654	52,654	50,000	50,000	200,000	4,500	7,200	73,477	254,359	335,177	**589,536**
Chargeback Service	-	91,562	91,562	123,000	10,000	-	-	-	-	306,124	10,000	**316,124**
Animal Supplies & Services	-	-	-	-	-	-	-	-	-	-	-	**-**
Travel	-	5,000	5,000	-	23,000	800	-	2,600	-	10,000	26,400	**36,400**
Other Scientific Expenses	-	-	-	-	40,000	-	-	-	-	-	40,000	**40,000**
Operational Expenses	6,332	6,167	6,167	38,059	10,000	83,000	16,000	16,500	-	56,725	125,500	**182,225**
Professional Fees	290	-	-	-	-	290	-	-	290	290	580	**870**
Other Expenses	25,400	187,679	187,679	46,193	13,500	6,500	300	600	-	446,951	20,900	**467,851**
Recruiting and Relocation	-	-	-	-	-	-	-	-	-	-	-	**-**
Information Technology	2,000	2,000	2,000	2,300	500	2,500	5,000	5,000	10,000	8,300	23,000	**31,300**
Total Costs	$ 511,734	$ 756,563	$ 863,471	$ 445,079	$ 387,380	$ 757,782	$ 44,907	$ 116,324	$ 211,060	$ 2,576,847	$ 1,517,452	**$4,094,299**
Total Net Budget (net of budgeted external rev.)	$ 2,290	$ 2,000	$ 2,000	$ 2,300	$ 382,380	$ 357,782	$ 44,907	$ 116,324	$ 211,060	**$ 8,590**	**$1,112,452**	**$1,121,042**

known amounts of clinical data are not as valuable as those with treatment and outcome data. In addition, biospecimens from rare diseases or significant cohorts of subject populations bring greater value than common and/or singlet biospecimens that may not represent a population of subjects well. Selling tissues and biospecimens on the basis of a commodity profit is not permissible in the United States,[14] but recouping the collecting, processing, and storage costs that went into making the resource available is acceptable. National networks like the NCI Cooperative Human Tissue Network (CHTN)[15] will distribute biospeci-

Table 9-2. Itemized Project A for the Annual Budget Sheet for a Biorepository

RESEARCH INSTITUTE
BUDGET FY 2014
TOTAL BUDGET SUMMARY

Account Number	DESCRIPTION	Project A: Biobank 1	Biobank3	Biobank 3	Biobank 4	Total Grants	Institution Funded	Total
	Total Direct External Revenue	$ 509,444	$ 754,563	$ 861,471	$ 442,779	$ 2,568,257	$ 5,000	**$ 2,573,257**
	Capital Equipment							
1500	Capital Equipment	66,500				66,500		**$ 66,500**
	Total Capital Equipment	$ 66,500	$ -	$ -	$ -	$ 66,500		**$ 66,500**
	Salaries & Wages							
4001	Salaries	243,875	321,485	335,341	144,943	1,045,644	164,648	**1,210,292**
4012	Part-time Wages	-	-	-	-	-	8,670	**8,670**
	27th Pay Period					-	6,586	**6,586**
	Available (short) for personnel on grants & contracts					-		**-**
	Total Salaries & Wages	$ 243,875	$ 321,485	$ 335,341	$ 144,943	$ 1,045,644	$ 179,904	**$ 1,225,548**
	Other Compensation							
4126	Cell Phone Stipend					-	7,500	**7,500**
4124	Adjunct Compensation (Contract labor)			89,173		89,173		**89,173**
	Total Other Compensation	$ -	$ -	$ 89,173	$ -	$ 89,173	$ 7,500	**$ 185,846**
	Benefits							
4399	Full-Time Benefits (28%)	68,285	90,016	93,895	40,584	292,780	44,368	**337,148**
4399	Part-Time Benefits (16%)					-		**-**
4399	Part-Time Benefits (8%)	-	-	-	-	-	694	**694**
	27th Pay Period					-	(6,586)	**(6,586)**
	Available (short) for personnel on grants & contracts					-		**-**
	Total Benefits	$ 68,285	$ 90,016	$ 93,895	$ 40,584	$ 292,780	$ 38,476	**$ 331,256**
	Equipment / Software							
4401	Lab Equipment					-	10,000	**10,000**
4402	Computer Hardware					-	2,500	**2,500**
4403	Software					-		**-**
4405	Software maintenance					-	2,000	**2,000**
4406	Other Office Equipment					-		**-**
	Total Equipment / Software	$ -	$ -	$ -	$ -	$ -	$ 14,500	**$ 14,500**
	Lab Supplies & Services							
4503	Chemicals					-		**-**
4504	Controlled Materials					-		**-**
4505	Cleaning Supplies					-		**-**
4506	Laboratory Supplies	99,051	52,654	52,654	50,000	254,359	35,000	**289,359**
4507	Biological Reagents					-	10,000	**10,000**
4523	Supply Store					-	5,000	**5,000**
	Total Lab Supplies & Services	$ 99,051	$ 52,654	$ 52,654	$ 50,000	$ 254,359	$ 50,000	**$ 304,359**
	Internal Chargeback Service							
4510	Histology		91,562	91,562	123,000	306,124	10,000	**316,124**
4520	Liquid Nitrogen Freezer					-		**-**
4611	Vivarium Animal Holding Services					-		**-**
4623	Cryopreservation					-		**-**
	Total Internal Chargeback Service	$ -	$ 91,562	$ 91,562	$ 123,000	$ 306,124	$ 10,000	**$ 316,124**
	Animal Supplies & Services							
4624	General Animal Supplies					-		**-**
4603	Animal Purchases					-		**-**
	Total Animal Supplies & Services	$ -	$ -	$ -	$ -	$ -		**$ -**
	Travel							
4702	Meals					-	3,000	**3,000**
4705	Lodging					-	6,000	**6,000**
4706	Transportation		5,000	5,000		10,000	10,000	**20,000**
4707	Foreign Meals / Lodging / Transportation					-		**-**
4708	Registration Fees					-	4,000	**4,000**
4799	Pre-travel Expenses					-		**-**
	Total Travel	$ -	$ 5,000	$ 5,000	$ -	$ 10,000	$ 23,000	**$ 33,000**
	Other Scientific Expenses							
4803	Library Services					-		**-**
4807	Resource Materials					-		**-**
4809	Publications / Reprints / Abstracts					-		**-**
4817	Scientific Purchased Services					-	40,000	**40,000**
	Total Other Scientific Expenses	$ -	$ -	$ -	$ -	$ -	$ 40,000	**$ 40,000**
	Operational Expenses							
5008	Service Maintenance Agreements	5,550	6,167	6,167	2,000	19,884		**19,884**
5010	Repair and Maintenance - Equipment					-	10,000	**10,000**
5017	Facilities Chargeback	782			36,059	36,841		**36,841**
	Total Operational Expenses	$ 6,332	$ 6,167	$ 6,167	$ 38,059	$ 56,725	$ 10,000	**$ 66,725**
	Professional Fees							
5272	Consulting	290				290		**290**
	Total Professional Fees	$ 290	$ -	$ -	$ -	$ 290		**$ 290**
	Other Expenses							
5207	Office Supplies					-	3,500	**3,500**
5209	Express Shipping	25,400	186,517	186,517	46,193	444,627	1,000	**445,627**
5210	Freight					-	1,000	**1,000**
5211	Subscriptions					-	1,000	**1,000**
5212	Professional Dues					-	7,000	**7,000**
5299	Miscellaneous		1,162	1,162		2,324		**2,324**
	Total Other Expenses	$ 25,400	$ 187,679	$ 187,679	$ 46,193	$ 446,951	$ 13,500	**$ 460,451**
	Recruiting and Relocation							
5236	Temporary Housing - Non Relocation					-		**-**
5501	Recruiting					-		**-**
5502	Relocation					-		**-**
	Total Recruiting and Relocation	$ -	$ -	$ -	$ -	$ -	$ -	**$ -**
	Information Technology							
5601	Telephone & Telecommunications	500	500	500	800	2,300	500	**2,800**
5603	Internet Services	1,500	1,500	1,500	1,500	6,000		**6,000**
	Total Information Technology	$ 2,000	$ 2,000	$ 2,000	$ 2,300	$ 8,300	$ 500	**$ 8,800**
	Total Costs	$ 511,734	$ 756,563	$ 863,471	$ 445,079	$ 2,576,847	$ 387,330	**$ 2,964,177**
	Shared Resources - Lab Supplies					-		**-**
	Total Costs including Shared	$ 511,734	$ 756,563	$ 863,471	$ 445,079	$ 2,576,847	$ 387,330	**$ 2,964,177**
	Total Net Budget (net of budgeted external rev.)	$ 2,290	$ 2,000	$ 2,000	$ 2,300	$ 8,589	$ 382,330	**$ 390,919**

Table 9-4. Cooperative Human Tissue Network Fees, 2014

Processing Fees	Since the CHTN is an NCI-supported resource, investigators are only charged a LOW processing fee for each sample to offset the costs of collecting, handling, and preparing the specimens in accordance with the detailed requirements of the investigator. A sample is defined as one processed piece of a specimen, regardless of the sample size or type of processing. Each investigator is also responsible for all shipping costs. Effective Apr. 2, 2012, the processing fees are as follows: ▪ $50.00 processing fee/sample for investigators located at ACADEMIC/GOVERNMENT LAB sites ▪ $150.00 processing fee/sample for investigators located at COMMERCIAL organizations
Additional Services	Additional services can be provided to investigators upon request. These fees are applicable to both academic and commercial investigators. Hematoxilyn-eosin (H&E) slide $7.00 Unstained slide $5.00 Stained slide from frozen section $7.00 First cut, unstained slide from frozen section $6.00 Each additional cut from frozen section $4.00 20-micron section $8.50 5-cut ribbon (of routine thickness) $8.00 Touch preps $4.50 RNA Quality Check (per sample) $100.00 Frozen tissue macrodissection $40.00
Chart Reviews	Investigators may request chart reviews for a minimal fee.
Shipping Charges	Shipping charges are the responsibility of the investigator and are determined by the courier utilized. This charge will vary according to the weight and priority status of the shipment.

Source: Cooperative Human Tissue Network (CHTN), National Cancer Institute (NCI).[15]

mens on a per-unit basis as shown in Table 9-4. Tissue aliquots cost $50.00, and fluids, such as serum or plasma, may cost less. Derivatives like DNA or RNA will cost more because of the additional costs of the time, effort, and materials used in their preparation. Other biorepositories may distribute biospecimens at little or no cost, if the resource has been developed by a federal grant or contract and if those who are awarded the biospecimens have qualified through an approved biospecimen use committee that has verified the science and funding of the investigator who is benefiting from the use of the biospecimens.[16] Institutional biorepositories should request payback charges, but the amount is to be determined by the institution; there is not a specific formula used by all institutions. The determination is set between the willingness of the institution to support the biorepository and the ability of the users to pay for the service. Like many marketed services, the rate is defined by the ease of access and wide usability, which, in the end, should provide institutional success in research and additional resource advantages to the access of funded opportunities.

Conclusion

In conclusion, appropriate and aggressive management of the biorepository can reduce its overall costs, but the cost–benefit evaluation must include the enormous value that the biorepository provides to the institution's research accomplishments.

References

1. Centers for Disease Control and Prevention. www.cdc.gov/. Accessed March 31, 2014.
2. National Heart Lung and Blood Institute. Biologic Specimen and Data Repository Information Coordinating Center (BioLINCC). https://biolincc.nhlbi.nih.gov/home/. Accessed March 31, 2014.
3. The Joint Pathology Center. www.jpc.capmed.mil/leadership.asp. Accessed March 31, 2014.
4. Coriell Cell Repositories. Coriell Institute for Medical Research. ccr.coriell.org/. 2009. Accessed March 31, 2014.
5. *Moore v Regents of University of California.* 793 P 2d 479 (Cal 1990).
6. *The Washington University v Catalona.* 437 F.Supp.2d 985 (Mo 2006).

7. *Greenberg v Miami Children's Hospital Research Inst, Inc.* 264 F Supp 2d 1064 (S D Fla 2003).
8. Specialty Accreditation Programs. College of American Pathologists. www.cap.org/apps/cap.portal?_nfpb=true&cntvwrPtlt_actionOverride=%2Fportlets%2FcontentViewer%2Fshow&_windowLabel=cntvwrPtlt&cntvwrPtlt%7BactionForm.contentReference%7D=laboratory_accreditation%2Flap_info%2Fspecialty.html&_state=maximized&_pageLabel=cntvwr. Accessed March 31, 2014.
9. Lunshof JE, Church GM, Prainsack B. Raw personal data: Providing access. *Science.* 2014; 343:373-374.
10. Couzin-Frankel J. Divulging DNA secrets of dead stirs debate. *Science.* 2014;343: 356-357.
11. International Society for Biological and Environmental Repositories (ISBER). 2012 best practices for repositories: collection, storage, retrieval and distribution of biological materials for research. *Biopreserv Biobank.* 2012:10(2):79-161. Also available at www.isber.org. Accessed March 31, 2014.
12. Self-assessment tool (SAT) for repositories. International Society for Biological and Environmental Repositories. http://www.isber.org/?page=SAT. Accessed March 31, 2014.
13. *NCI Best Practices for Biospecimen Resources.* Office of Biorepositories and Biospecimen Research, National Cancer Institute. biospecimens.cancer.gov/bestpractices/. Accessed March 31, 2014.
14. National Organ Transplant Act. Public Law 98-507, 98 Stat. 2339-2348 (Oct. 19, 1984).
15. Processing fees. Cooperative Human Tissue Network, National Cancer Institute. www.chtn.nci.nih.gov/fees/. Accessed March 31, 2014.
16. Processing fees. Cooperative Group Banks, Biorepositories for NCI-Sponsored Cancer Clinical Trials. National Cancer Institute. cgb.cancer.gov/biospecimens/fees.html/. Accessed March 31, 2014.

Chapter 10

Relationships With Outside Institutions and Industry

Kimberly Myers
Nicole Lockhart

Perception of Sale of Tissue

The present framework for organ and biospecimen donation was born out of scandal. In 1827 and 1828 in Edinburgh, Scotland, William Burke and William Hare murdered 16 people in order to sell the cadavers for dissection in anatomy lectures.[1] Burke was subsequently executed for his crimes in front of a large crowd, and his cadaver was used in an anatomy lecture the following day.[1] A pocketbook made from Burke's tanned skin is on display at the Surgeons' Hall Museum, Royal College of Surgeons of Edinburgh.[2] The use of human bodies for medical science became a significant public issue after this incident and led to the creation of the Anatomy Act of the United Kingdom in 1832.[3] This act allowed for the provision of cadavers from hospitals, work houses, and prisons *only* if the bodies were unclaimed.[3] The Anatomy Act set the initial tone and shaped the thinking that one cannot sell or put a price on a body. It provided a reason to stay with the gifting framework—avoidance of murder, mutilation, and theft of bodies.

The rise of autonomy in American law and bioethics further shaped the public's attitude about the property status of the body. When organ transplantation involving living persons emerged in the 1950s, it engendered heated controversy over its morality. Concerns ranged from objections to mutilation of the human body, even to save another life; fear that donors would be exploited and feel obligated to donate; and opposition to the possible commodification of the human body. In order to protect potential donors from these moral hazards, the Uniform Anatomical Gift Act supports the requirement for informed and voluntary donation and prohibits trafficking in human organs.[4] Respect for persons through informed consent continues to be a key ethical principle recognized both in the *The Belmont Report*[5] and in the Common Rule,[6] which governs research conducted or supported by the US Department of Health and Human Services and other federal agencies.

The perception of profit from human biospecimens obtained without proper consent for research or without disclosure of the intent to develop commercial products has led to multiple lawsuits in the United States. In the case of *Moore v Regents of the University of California* (1990), the patient, John Moore, sued his physician and the University of California after discovering that a cell line derived from his blood and tissues was being patented.[7] Moore was under the impression that his specimens were needed only for his clinical care and was unaware that any research was being conducted with his specimens.[7] Although the California Supreme Court ruled that Moore did not have property rights to a new product developed from his tissues because the product was "factually and legally distinct" from his excised cells, the Court also ruled that Moore's physician had breached his fiduciary duty by failing to disclose research and economic interests in Moore's tissue during the informed consent process.[7] In the case of *Greenberg v Miami Children's Hospital* (2003), a group of individuals and nonprofit organizations donated specimens and genetic information to a well-known researcher in the hopes of expediting the isolation of the gene associated with Canavan disease.[8] When the researcher subsequently patented the genetic sequence for Canavan disease and the research institution began negotiating exclusive licenses and charging royalty fees for Canavan disease testing, two parents of children with Canavan disease as well as several other parties sued the researcher and the research institution, alleging, among other claims, breach of informed consent, breach of fiduciary duty, and unjust enrichment.[8] Although the majority of the plaintiffs' claims ultimately were dismissed, the claim for unjust enrichment was upheld in recognition of the significant contribution of time and money made by the plaintiffs.[8]

The Moore and Greenberg cases are most often cited in relation to the ownership of human tissue, but both cases also highlight the importance of disclosing any commercial intent to research participants during the informed consent process. In both cases, the suits brought by the patients were at least partially motivated by the fact that, as research participants, these patients had no knowledge of the researcher's intention to develop commercial products, with potential profits, from their donated specimens. The need to address whether biospecimens and/or data may be used by for-profit entities and the possible development of downstream commercial products has been stressed in National Cancer Institute (NCI) recommendations related to informed consent.[9,10] In addition, the American Medical Association Code of Ethics states that "human tissue and its products may not be used for commercial purposes without the informed consent of the patient who provided the original cellular material."[11] Several model informed-consent documents for biospecimen donation explicitly state that whereas biospecimens will not be sold, they may be used by commercial entities to develop new treatments or products, and biospecimen donors will not be compensated or receive any portion of future profits[12] (eg, The Cancer Genome Atlas [TCGA],[13] and Public Population Project in Genomics [P3G][14] model consents). When members of the public representative of potential biospecimen donors were asked how they would feel if commercial products were developed from specimens they donated, about one-third of interviewees felt positive about the development of commercial products and another third were comfortable with this concept; however, about one fifth of interviewees responded negatively to the possibility that researchers could profit from specimens or data that they donated.[15] Even though the majority of research participants appear to support development of commercial products from biospecimens, any intended commercial use should be disclosed in the informed consent document in order to promote transparency and ensure that donors fully understand and agree to the proposed use(s) of their biospecimens.

The increasing importance of the use of biospecimens in research has raised awareness of the key role of human research participants in the research process and, accordingly, has brought the issue of benefit sharing to the forefront. In this context, the term *benefit sharing* refers to sharing the financial or nonfinancial rewards realized from human specimen research with the research participants who made the research possible in the first place or with humankind more broadly.[16] The idea that at least some form of benefit sharing is morally appropriate has been endorsed widely by international health organizations (the World Health Organization[17] and the Human Genome Organisation [HUGO][18]) and specific disease groups. The 2012 edition of the International Society for Biological and Environmental Repositories (ISBER) *Best Practices for Repositories* states, "Repositories that import specimens and data from other countries should respect the autonomy of the providing country and ensure that fair and equitable benefits are made available to the providing country."[19] The questions of if and how benefits should be shared with biospecimen donors in less-developed countries is particularly controversial and has led to some countries implementing more stringent requirements for the export of biospecimens for research.[20]

Benefit sharing need not be limited to profit sharing or other forms of financial compensation. Nonfinancial benefits, such as health-related research results, could also serve as a potential benefit to interested research participants. In a survey of parents of children and adolescents with cancer in the United States and Canada, Fernandez et al[21,22] reported that more than 90% of participants in each group felt that they have a strong right to be informed of research results from a clinical trial in which they participated. Similarly, Partridge et al[23,24] found that 96% of women with breast cancer participating in a phase II trial felt that they have a right to the research results; 90% chose to be provided with the research results when offered. Although return of individual research results remains controversial because of concerns about analytic validity and clinical utility,[25] return of aggregate or summary-level research results demonstrates respect for research participants, with lower risk of harm due to inaccurate findings or misinterpreted clinical significance. The 2007 NCI workshop "Custodianship and Ownership Issues in Biospecimen Research" resulted in the following recommendation: "Clear and specific informed consent language should be used to ensure that those who contribute biospecimens and/or data for research purposes comprehend any financial or nonfinancial benefits they may receive from the products, tests, or discoveries resulting from the research."[9] While provision of research results or other benefits may not be possible in all cases, researchers must ensure that biospecimen contributors have a clear understanding of how their specimens will be used and whether they are likely to receive any benefits as a result of their participation.

In addition to disclosing any intended commercial use of biospecimens and any potential benefits to participants during the informed consent process, biorepositories should also consider use of a Material Transfer Agreement (MTA) or other appropriate agreement to prevent downstream research uses that may conflict with the informed consent provided by the research participant or the stated purpose of the biobank. As the primary agreement between the biobank and the end user, the MTA serves as the best mechanism for documenting acceptable and prohibited uses of the biospecimens as well as the corresponding responsibilities of the two parties. Relevant terms in such agreements generally prohibit transfer of specimens/data to third parties without explicit prior approval from the biobank/provider, direct sale of biospecimens or derivatives (eg, DNA or protein isolated from the biospecimens), and attempted reidentification of biospecimen contributors by the recipient. In addition, the agreement may specify the biobank's policy regarding patenting of biospecimens or their derivatives by end users. Several model MTAs are publicly available and may be adapted to meet the specific needs of an individual biobank (eg, National Cancer Institute *NCI Best Practices for Biospecimen Resources*,[10] Uniform Biological Material Transfer Agreement,[26] Cooperative Human Tissue Network Agreement for Use of Tissue,[27] National Institutes of Health Office of Technology Transfer[28]).

Oversight of Agreements With Industry or Other Parties

Appropriate and transparent mechanisms for oversight of a biobank are essential to ensuring public trust and overall quality operations. The Office for Human Research Protections has issued guidance that biorepositories conducting nonexempt human subjects research should be subject to oversight by an Institutional Review Board (IRB).[29] As described in the guidance, the IRB should review and approve a protocol specifying the conditions under which data and specimens may be accepted and shared and ensure adequate provisions to protect the privacy of subjects and maintain the confidentiality of data.[29] The IRB should also review and approve a sample collection protocol and informed consent document for distribution to tissue collectors and their local IRBs. NCI recommendations also support a clearly established governance and oversight structure consisting of the set of authorities, processes, and procedures guiding key operational decisions made within the resource.[10] Governance affects access and research use decisions and custodial relationships and responsibilities. Specifically, the most current version of the NCI Best Practices recommends that the following issues be addressed in the governance plan[10]:

> (1) How does the biospecimen resource propose to ensure the physical integrity of biospecimens? (2) How does the biospecimen resource propose to ensure the integrity of the human research participant data that accompany the biospecimens? (3) What plans and protocols are in place for the distribution of samples to investigators? (4) What are the roles and responsibilities of the biospecimen resource director and his or her institution?

The NCI Best Practices further recommends that biospecimen resources develop a legacy or contingency plan as part of the overall governance plan.[10] The legacy plan should address the handling and disposition of biospecimens and associated data at one or more of the following points: (1) end of the budget period of the grant, (2) loss of management or termination of funding, (3) accomplishment of the specific research objectives of the study, (4) depletion of biospecimens, (5) achievement of critical data end points, and/or (6) discontinuation of participation by human research participants.[10] Any special relationships or privileges, such as preferred access to biospecimens or data by a particular group, should be described in the governance plan as well as any oversight mechanisms which monitor such relationships. The governance structure should be described either in the informed consent document or in supplementary materials to ensure that research participants understand the mechanisms to protect their privacy and confidentiality and under what conditions researchers will be able to gain access to their specimens and data.[10] Disclosure of biobank governance and oversight models may be considered particularly important if research participants are asked to provide broad consent for future research. In such cases, the governance and oversight structure serves as the primary means of ensuring that participants' specimens and data are used appropriately because the participant is unable to specify preferred uses for his or her specimen. In the interest of transparency, biobanks should consider making their governance structure public through posting on the Internet or via other mechanisms, as has been done for some high-profile biobanks.[30]

Access to Biospecimens and Data

Perhaps the most contentious issue surrounding biorepositories is how access to biospecimens will be granted and which parties will have priority access to specimens and/or data. An analysis of publicly available access policies for biorepositories associated with population science identified nine key elements: (1) the existence of a Data Access Committee (DAC); (2) a timeline for collaboration; (3) criteria for evaluating proposed ancillary studies; (4) publicly available information about the host study; (5) cost-recovery plans; (6) considerations of human subject and intellectual property issues; (7) information on the handling of the biospecimen; (8) guidelines for publications, presentations, and credit; and (9) a process for resolving disputes.[31]

While the analysis by Lemrow et al[31] was specific to population biobanks, several of the elements will be the same or similar for disease-based biobanks. Both the NCI Best Practices[28] and the ISBER Best Practices[19] include more detailed recommendations regarding the evaluation of access proposals, including such factors as scientific merit, statistical validity, qualifications of the requesting investigator, and impact of the proposed research. In addition, both sets of best practices stress the importance of transparent access policies and consistency with the informed consent provided by the original research participants.[10,19]

Transparent access policies should include not only the criteria by which applications will be judged, but also a clear description of whether any parties will have priority access to specimens or data. In some cases, priority or preferred access may be appropriate; for example, if the specimens or data were collected for a primary study, there may be a need to ensure that any ancillary studies are consistent with and complementary to the original study.[31] Alternatively, if specimens were collected with government funding, it may be appropriate to allow other government-funded projects to have priority (Cooperative Human Tissue Network Investigator Application Requirements and Priority).[27] Any exception to the general access policy and process for review, such as preferred access to funders of the biobank, should be explicitly noted. Biobank managers or others who make access decisions should also be aware of both real and perceived conflicts of interest. Financial conflicts of interest may arise if those funding the biobank are given preferred access to specimens without having to adhere to the same scientific standards of other investigators. Nonfinancial conflicts of interest may also arise, such as in situations where the individual managing the biobank is also a researcher seeking access to biospecimens.[10] Any financial or nonfinancial conflicts of interest should be publicly disclosed, for example on the biobank website or in the informed consent document or accompanying materials.[10] At a minimum, the informed consent document should contain a brief description of the types of researchers who will have access to the specimens and the process for review and/or the oversight for the access process.

Researchers and biobank managers must ensure that access to biospecimens corresponds with the research participant's wishes and intentions as described in the informed consent document. Cases in which biospecimens were perceived to be used in a manner inconsistent with or beyond the scope of the original consent have led research participants to sue researchers and their institutions. In 1990, members of the Havasupai tribe donated blood samples to researchers from Arizona State University with the understanding that the samples would be used to study the high incidence of diabetes in the tribe.[32,33] The samples were subsequently used for wide-ranging studies including research related to schizophrenia and theories of the tribe's geographical origins that contradicted their traditional beliefs.[32,33] In April 2010, the Arizona State University Board of Regents settled a lawsuit brought by members of the Havasupai and agreed to pay $700,000 to 41 of the tribe's members, return the blood samples, and provide other forms of assistance to the impoverished Havasupai, such as scholarships and assistance in obtaining money for a new health clinic.[32,33] In the Havasupai case, consent was obtained for the original biospecimen collection; however, research participants did not think that they were adequately informed about how their samples may be used in the future or that additional researchers would be able to access them for new studies without the approval of the tribe.[32,33]

In other cases, litigation has resulted from the use of biospecimens obtained in the course of clinical care and used for research without the knowledge of research participants. Parents in Texas sued the state health agency after a reporter tipped them off to the fact that dried blood spots used for state-mandated newborn screening were being made available to scientists for research without authorization from the families.[34] Some samples had even been provided to federal law enforcement officials for research to improve forensic DNA evidence.[34] The state ultimately settled the case and destroyed all 5.3 million blood samples.[35]

As demonstrated by these high-profile cases, research participants care deeply about both the types of research that will be performed, as well as who will have access to their samples. They expect that all material information will be presented to them and that their samples will not be used without their consent. Although in many cases biospecimens are collected for the purpose of establishing a biobank for broad future research, it is still vital to describe what types of research will and will not be allowed, as well as how access will be granted, in order to prevent future misunderstandings. In general, most empirical studies have shown a willingness of research participants to consent for use of biospecimens for research, with the percent willing ranging from 80% to 95%.[36] The majority of participants are even comfortable with broad consent for unspecified research, but they do want and expect to be asked for their consent.[36]

Intellectual Property and Authorship Policies

Because of the fundamental role that biospecimens play in research and development, significant advances may arise using biospecimens acquired from outside institutions. Many advances, such as technology, diagnostics, and therapeutics development, may have commercial potential and therefore intellectual property value. Transactions involving intellectual property have great implications for both parties involved,[37] as well as for the general public. These implications include a public-good benefit through the development of marketable products and also an impact on the US economy's growth and development. In addition, authorship concerns, particularly in academic institutions, may exist.

It has become increasingly important for biobanks to establish mechanisms for addressing intellectual property concerns. Robust intellectual property and data sharing policies should be developed and shared widely with customers and partnering organizations. Significant effort should be devoted to developing authorship and intellectual property policies that are consistent with local, state, and federal regulations. Many National Institutes of Health (NIH) policies address these issues and should be referred to while creating institutional intellectual property and data sharing policies. The NCI Best Practices[10] outlines the following issues that should be addressed in the development of intellectual property and data sharing policies for a biobank (also see section in Best Practices on Material Transfer Agreements):

- What, if any, rights do recipients have to further distribute the biospecimens?
- Are there assurances of end users' right to publish research results and findings?
- Intellectual property terms should be consistent with the NIH Research Tools Policy[38] and other applicable NIH sharing policies.[39]
- What, if any, conditions or limitations exist on commercial use?
- What, if any, expectations exist for the dissemination of research data?
- The resource should provide a clear description of the biospecimens and/or unmodified derivatives covered by the agreement.

Some biobanks may request or require that recipients return molecular analysis data about acquired biospecimens back to the resource. In addition, some publicly funded biobanks may require sharing of results and supporting information. For example, the UK Biobank, supported by both public and private funds, requires the deposit of all results from analysis on participant samples and participant data into the UK Biobank database.[30,40] The NIH maintains a data sharing policy that requires researchers to have a data sharing plan for grant applications greater than $500,000.[41] *NCI Best Practices for Biospecimen Resources*[10] advises that research data and research resources obtained using biospecimens should be made available to the research community to the greatest extent possible, consistent with, as applicable, the NIH Data Sharing Policy,[42] other applicable NIH sharing policies,[39] and the NIH Research Tools Policy.[38]

Recognizing the need for industry researchers to develop new drugs and products based on their findings and the need for academic and other researchers to produce publications based on their findings, biobanks must work to establish data sharing policies that honor both the value of biospecimens housed in a biobank and the need for end users to protect their research findings, while also contributing to the public good. As such, if a biobank requires the return of data, it should proactively establish and document, in an MTA or similar agreement, what data should be returned to the resource and in what time frame. The time frame for the return of data should allow for a limited period of exclusivity to allow end users to publish and/or pursue intellectual property rights for research conducted using the biospecimens.

In the absence of a greater scientific contribution, the collection, processing, and storage of biospecimens (which are activities generally performed by the biobank staff) generally do not constitute inventorship on patents as it is defined by US patent law; however, inventorship is determined by law and must be evaluated on a case-by-case basis.[10] In addition, the biobank generally will retain no rights to intellectual property generated by third-party biospecimen end users.[10] Such policies should be clearly outlined in intellectual property and data sharing policies and in MTAs.

When a biobank is federally funded and supported, the Bayh-Dole Act[43] (also known as the Patent and Trademark Law Amendments Act) provides key ground rules and regulations for relationships involving the generation of intellectual property. Passed in 1980, the Bayh-Dole Act applies to large and small businesses, universities, and nonprofit organizations and creates a uniform policy to deal with inventions arising from research supported by federal dollars.[37] Perhaps the most significant provision of the Bayh-Dole Act is that it gives universities control over intellectual property generated using federally provided research dollars. Institutions funded by federal dollars can elect ownership in their inventions and have the right to further develop and commercialize these products. In addition, such institutions can license the invention to third parties. An important consequence of this provision is that it provides strong incentives for universities to establish research collaborations with industry.[44]

Under the Bayh-Dole Act, if the federal government determines that a product is not being made available for the public good on a reasonable basis, the government can exercise "march-in" rights to license the product to third parties. March-in rights do not require the consent of the patent holder or original licensee. Federal agencies, such as the NIH, may periodically audit for compliance with the Bayh-Dole Act.[44] Under certain circumstances, a federal agency can determine that the federal government should hold the ownership of the invention. In such cases, the decision must be made before entering into the funding agreement, and the federal agency must file a "Determination of Exceptional Circumstances" with the Department of Commerce.

Partnering to Create Sustainable Resources

Historically, biobanking and the formation of biobanks have developed in a "siloed" fashion, with individual investigators and institutions developing their own biobanks to meet specific research needs.[45] As a result, a lack of standardization and harmonization between research institutions exists. Such individual approaches to biobanking often result in inconsistent funding and resources limited to only those that an individual researcher or institution can provide.[45] Biobanks are resource-intense operations, requiring considerable expertise to develop standard operating procedures; obtain informed consent from patients; address ethical, legal, and policy concerns; procure and process patient samples; manage quality; and ensure access.[46] The cost of maintaining multiple unshared resources will generally exceed that of maintaining a single shared resource. Furthermore, the ability of outside institutions to gain access to biobanks at other institutions has proved problematic and has the effect of limiting both collaboration and the advancement of translational research.

In a time of significant financial investment in biomedical research, many stakeholders have been frustrated by a perceived slow or low return on investment in research.[47] Alternative and more efficient funding methods are being considered as potential solutions to some concerns. Partnerships allow organizations to leverage intellectual and financial investments that contribute to the success of biobanking initiatives. Although perception issues and access concerns can be complex, partnering with outside institutions can often help to create access to diverse populations of biospecimens and to create transparency and trust, both within the scientific community and with the general public. New partnership models between public organizations (such as federal and state governments) and private entities (such as research and patient advocacy groups, universities, biotechnology companies, and pharmaceutical companies) may create opportunities that foster the public trust and enable rapid advancement of translational research through the use of biobanking resources.

Partnerships may take numerous forms, with a vast array of options for types of partnering organizations and governance and operational models. Some institutions may prefer to partner with similar organizations (ie, advocacy organizations partnering with other advocacy organizations to address specific needs). Such relationships are most often established because of clear synergy in the goals of the partnering institutions. As such, these alliances may prove to be easier and less complex to launch. However, organizations may find that these relationships are limited and limiting because they do not have a diverse knowledge base and expertise from different types of organizations.

There is recent movement toward establishing public–private partnerships to support translational research.[48] These relationships generally involve one or more state or federal government institutions working with one or more private organizations, including academia, industry, research, and patient advocacy organizations. These relationships allow the public and private sectors to create infrastructures that neither sector possesses the resources on its own to achieve.[49] The merits of establishing a partnering relationship must be measured against several criteria, including an evaluation of the risks and benefits to each party, an evaluation of each party's future ability to afford to sustain its role in the partnership, and an understanding of the social benefits derived in context of the moneys committed by the partnering organizations.[49]

Creating partnerships and business models that organize diverse stakeholders around common infrastructure presents opportunities for great rewards, but also great challenges.[50] Before such a resource can be embraced by all relevant stakeholders, questions of access, governance, and transparency need to be addressed. The following questions become apparent when considering a collaborative biobanking model:

- What are the specific roles of each partner?
- What incentives exist for participation in a shared resource?[50]

- How do you ensure an environment of trust and transparency among partners? What resources are available to earn and ensure the public trust?
- How are costs distributed among partners?[50]
- How do you develop robust access, intellectual property, custodianship, and data sharing policies that are beneficial and transparent to all parties and that all parties can agree upon?
- Should access to samples be restricted to only partnering organizations? What are the access policies and what are the restrictions?[46]
- Will samples be provided free of charge to partners or outside institutions? If not, at what price?[46]

Recent discussions about biobanking partnerships at the NCI yielded several "lessons learned" from other biobanking initiatives. Several factors were cited as common among successful biobanking initiatives, regardless of the funding structure, governance structure, or location of the biobank[49]:

- Custodianship issues must be addressed proactively.
- Transparency is essential to building trust among partners.
- Insurance of quality and supply is critical to partner participation.
- In general, some level of government support is essential to sustainability.[51] This is probably a function of the resource and cost-intensive nature of biobanking enterprises.

Federal agencies, particularly the NIH, have realized the important role that biobanks play in driving translational research and personalized medicine.[50] In response, the NIH has produced biobank guidelines such as the *NCI Best Practices for Biospecimen Resources*.[10] An emphasis on harmonizing practices, and the support and regulation of ethical policies and procedures, may make the timing right for the federal government to take on the role of both managing and funding key biobanks. Several countries and international bodies, including the European Union, the United Kingdom, Singapore, and Luxembourg, are currently building or operating national biobanks. However, tight budgetary constraints at agencies such as the NIH do not allow the government to be the sole funding source in such initiatives. Furthermore, the most effective models for a public-good structure would also need to be highly transparent. With that in mind, the presence of other nongovernmental organizations and stakeholders in the decision-making process could be essential to the success of national biobanking initiatives.

Advocates and advocacy organizations are recognizing the importance of biospecimens in research. Organizations such as the Lance Armstrong Foundation and the Multiple Myeloma Research Foundation have begun to raise funds to implement plans to create their own biobanks.[52] Patient advocacy organizations have many strengths—disease area expertise, an understanding of cost structures and models, efficiency management, and close contact with the public—that could place them in a strong strategic position to realize the vision and success of biobank initiatives. Many advocacy organizations, however, may find that they lack either the scientific expertise or the financial resources to start and run a biobank on their own. For those organizations, the possibility of partnering with public and private entities and working together to serve broad research needs could be appealing.

Biospecimen availability and quality have significant impacts on the ability of private companies to bring products to market, as well as on the time and expense associated with doing so. For example, human biospecimens are used by biotechnology and pharmaceutical companies to identify therapeutic targets and define molecular corollaries.[53] Human biospecimens are often used as a preclinical intermediate between the use of animal models and human clinical therapeutic trials.[53] Depending on the need, and often at significant expense, companies may develop their own biobanks or rely on external contracts to collect and gain access to biospecimens. During periods of declining revenues in the private sector, industry may be interested in partnership models that increase rapid access to high-quality diseased and normal biospecimens, decrease costs associated with acquiring and using biospecimens, and increase patient accrual into clinical research.

Alliances to fund and maintain biobanks also come with risks to each partner. From the advocacy perspective, issues such as patient consent and privacy protections would need to be addressed. Prioritizing the types of disease biospecimens to collect and quantities needed could prove to be difficult points of negotiation in creating a biobank with the involvement of different disease-specific advocacy communities. One significant obstacle for industry would be if the model required data sharing among partners and the intellectual property rights issues that could result. A partnership model involving industry would need to consider creative ways to make investment in shared resources appealing from financial and business investment points of view. For example, in order to obtain a waiver for data sharing requirements, industry may be more willing to pay higher biospecimen access fees or contribute more to the costs of building and maintaining the physical structure of the biobank.

Any institutional collaborative model will require a governance structure that represents the needs of all partnering organizations.[45] The manner in which this structure is set up and operates will be different from group to group, but the following key issues should be addressed:

- **Structure and representation.** Numerous models, including boards, executive teams, and so forth, exist for structuring and governing the partnership. The method should be agreed upon by all partnering organizations. Each partnering organization should have its interests represented within the governance model. Representation of diverse subject matter experts—covering such areas as scientific, economic, and policy expertise—will enable the organization to address the variety of issues that may arise.
- **Priority setting.** Priority setting for a collaborative model is a significant challenge, especially when stakeholders represent disparate interests. The governance structure should have a mechanism for establishing scientific priorities and resolving conflict. Access, data sharing, long-term custodianship, and intellectual property policies should be firmly in place and agreed upon by all involved parties.
- **Adherence to local, federal and state regulations.**[45] The governing body must ensure that all ethical, legal, and policy frameworks are adhered to and that any additional policies put in place by the collaboration are recognized.

Regardless of the final, agreed-upon structure, a strong outreach and education strategy for both the partnering institutions and the potential participants (ie, the public) would aid in overcoming perception concerns. In this case, open communication and transparency may aid the general public's understanding and acceptance of biobanking resources and facilitate a more engaged public in tissue contribution. For example, the resource may consider publishing a regular newsletter that informs participants of aggregate research results, including publications, therapeutics, and inventions resulting from the use of banked specimens. In an age of social media, the resource should consider nontraditional communication vehicles to aid its efforts. "Real-time" reports via blogs and the online community can help to actively engage the public in emerging research and the public's contribution to that process.

A process that engages all stakeholders early and solicits their input about biospecimen collection, access, and use may serve to overcome any perceived problems. Although partnering models for producing shared biobanks generate many questions that require careful thought and planning, the opportunity to bring diverse stakeholder groups together has unique benefits. Capitalizing on the expertise and shared financing from government, other nonprofit, and for-profit organizations would create structures that benefit multiple research enterprises. In addition, a model that generates broad access to biospecimens could maximize both the scientific and economic value of biospecimen collection and storage, while contributing to the public good.

Conclusion

As both the demand for biospecimens and the level of required quality increase, biobanks may need to consider alternative models of operation, including relationships with industry and other organizations, such as advocacy groups. Such partnerships may allow biobanks to reduce costs through increased efficiency and capitalize on diverse expertise from various partners. In order to make such relationships successful, policies must be completely transparent in terms of the nature of the relationship and the expectations of all parties. Issues such as intellectual property, access policies, and governance must be addressed before and during the formation of such relationships. Research participants must be fully informed about how such relationships may affect the use of their biospecimen sample. In addition, any obligations to the research participant must be honored.

References

1. MacDonald H. *Human Remains: Dissection and Its Histories.* New Haven, CT: Yale University Press; 2006.
2. Royal College of Surgeons of Edinburgh. Surgeons' Hall Museum. http://www.museum.rcsed.ac.uk/content/content.aspx?ID=33. Accessed March 31, 2014.
3. MacDonald H. Procuring corpses: the English anatomy inspectorate, 1842 to 1858. *Med Hist.* 2009;53(3):379-396.
4. Anatomical Gift Act (2006). Uniform Law Commission. The National Conference of Commissioners on Uniform State Laws. http://www.uniformlaws.org/Act.aspx?title=Anatomical%20Gift%20Act%20(2006). Accessed March 31, 2014.
5. The National Commission for the Protection of Hu- National Commission for the Protection of Human Subjects of Biomedical and Behavioral Research. *The Belmont Report. Ethical Principles and Guidelines for the Protection of Human Subjects of Research.* Washington, DC: National Institutes of Health, Department

of Health, Education, and Welfare, Office of Human Subjects Research; April 18, 1979. http://www.hhs.gov/ohrp/humansubjects/guidance/belmont.html. Accessed March 31, 2014.
6. US Department of Health and Human Services. Protection of Human Subjects ("Common Rule"). 45 CFR §46. http://www.hhs.gov/ohrp/humansubjects/guidance/45cfr46.html. Revised January 15, 2009. Effective July 14, 2009. Accessed March 31, 2014.
7. *Moore v Regents of University of California*. 793 P 2d 479 (Cal 1990).
8. *Greenberg v Miami Children's Hospital Research Inst, Inc.* 264 F Supp 2d 1064 (S D Fla 2003).
9. Office of Biorepositories and Biospecimen Research, National Cancer Institute. *Custodianship and Ownership Issues in Biospecimen Research: Summary.* National Institutes of Health, US Department of Health and Human Services. http://biospecimens.cancer.gov/resources/publications/workshop/cow.asp. Published May 2008. Accessed March 31, 2014.
10. Office of Biorepositories and Biospecimen Research, National Cancer Institute. *NCI Best Practices for Biospecimen Resources.* Washington, DC: National Institutes of Health, US Department of Health and Human Services; 2011. http://biospecimens.cancer.gov/practices/2011bp.asp. Accessed March 31, 2014.
11. AMA Code of Medical Ethics. Opinion 2.08: Commercial use of human tissue. American Medical Association. http://www.ama-assn.org/ama/pub/physician-resources/medical-ethics/code-medical-ethics/opinion208.page. Accessed March 31, 2014.
12. Beskow LM, Friedman JY, Hardy NC, Lin L, Weinfurt KP. Developing a simplified consent form for biobanking. PLoS One. 2010;5(10):e13302.
13. The Cancer Genome Atlas (TCGA): Informed consent documents. National Cancer Institute. http://cancergenome.nih.gov/abouttcga/policies/informedconsent. Accessed March 31, 2014.
14. Genetics and Society Project. Montreal University. Model Consent Form. Public Population Project in Genomics. 2007. http://www.p3gobservatory.org/repository/ethics.htm. Accessed March 31, 2014.
15. Beskow LM, Dean E. Informed consent for biorepositories: assessing prospective participants' understanding and opinions. *Cancer Epidemiol Biomarkers Prev.* 2008;17(6):1440-1451.
16. Pullman D, Latus A. Clinical trials, genetic add-ons, and the question of benefit-sharing. *Lancet.* 2002;362:242-244.
17. Report of a WHO Meeting on Collaboration in Medical Genetics. Toronto, Canada, April 9-10, 2002. World Health Organization Human Genetics Programme, 2002. http://whqlibdoc.who.int/hq/2002/WHO_HGN_WG_02.2.pdf. Accessed April 5, 2013.
18. Ethics Committee, Human Genome Organization. Statement on Benefit-Sharing. World Health Organization. http://www.who.int/genomics/elsi/regulatory_data/region/international/043/en/index.html. Accessed April 5, 2013.
19. International Society for Biological and Environmental Repositories (ISBER). 2012 best practices for repositories: collection, storage, retrieval and distribution of biological materials for research. *Biopreserv Biobank.* 2012:10(2):79-161. Also available at www.isber.org. Accessed March 31, 2014.
20. Office for Human Research Protections. International Compilation of Human Research Standards. 2013 Edition. US Department of Health and Human Services. http://www.hhs.gov/ohrp/international/index.html. Accessed April 4, 2013.
21. Fernandez CV, Taweel S, Kodish ED, Weijer C. Disclosure of research results to research participants: a pilot study of the needs and attitudes of adolescents and parents. *Paediatr Child Health.* 2005;10(6):332-334.
22. Fernandez CV, Gao J, Strahlendorf C, et al. Providing research results to participants: attitudes and needs of adolescents and parents of children with cancer. *J Clin Oncol.* 2009;27(6):878-883.
23. Partridge AH, Burstein HJ, Gelman RS, Marcom PK, Winer EP. Do patients participating in clinical trials want to know study results? *J Natl Cancer Inst.* 2003; 95(6):491-492.
24. Partridge AH, Wong JS, Knudsen K, et al. Offering participants results of a clinical trial: sharing results of a negative study. *Lancet.* 2005;365(9463):963-964.
25. Dressler LG. Disclosure of research results from cancer genomic studies: state of the science. *Clin Cancer Res.* 2009;15(13):4270-4276.
26. Uniform Biological Material Transfer Agreement. http://www.stanford.edu/group/ICO/researchAdmins/documents/ubmta_000.pdf. Accessed April 4, 2013.
27. Cooperative Human Tissue Network. Investigator Application Requirements and Priority. CHTN Application. National Cancer Institute. http://chtn.nci.nih.gov/requirements/. Accessed April 4, 2013.
28. Office of Technology Transfer. Forms and Model Agreements. National Institutes of Health, US Department of Health and Human Services. http://www.ott.nih.gov/forms_model_agreements/forms_model_agreements.aspx. Accessed April 4, 2013.
29. Office for Protection from Research Risks. Issues to Consider in the Research Use of Stored Data or Tissues. US Department of Health and Human Services. http://www.hhs.gov/ohrp/policy/reposit.html. Published November 7, 1997. Accessed March 31, 2014.
30. UK Biobank Ethics and Governance Framework. Version 3.0 (October 2007). http://www.ukbiobank.ac.uk/wp-content/uploads/2011/05/EGF20082.pdf. Accessed March 31, 2014.
31. Lemrow SM, Colditz GA, Vaught JB, Hartge P. Key elements of access policies for biorepositories associated with population science research. *Cancer Epidemiol Biomarkers Prev.* 2007;16(8):1533-1535.
32. Harmon A. Indian tribe wins fight to limit research of its DNA. *New York Times.* April 21, 2010.
33. Mello MM, Wolf LE. The Havasupai Indian tribe case: lessons for research involving stored biologic samples. *N Engl J Med.* 2010;363(3):204–207.

34. Harmon A. Where'd you go with my DNA? *New York Times.* April 23, 2010. http://www.nytimes.com/2010/04/22/us/22dna.html?pagewanted=all&_r=0. Accessed April 15, 2013.
35. Statement: Newborn Screening Settlement. Texas Department of State Health Services. News Release, December 22, 2009. http://www.dshs.state.tx.us/news/releases/20091222.shtm. Accessed April 4, 2013.
36. Wendler D. One-time general consent for research on biological samples. *BMJ.* 2006;332(7540):544-547.
37. Brock JL Jr. *Intellectual Property: Industry and Agency Concerns over Intellectual Property Rights.* Testimony: Before the Subcommittee on Technology and Procurement Policy, Committee on Government Reform, House of Representatives. May 10, 2002. US General Accounting Office. GAO-02-723T. www.gao.gov/new.items/d02723t.pdf. Accessed March 31, 2014.
38. National Institutes of Health. US Department of Health and Human Services. Principles and guidelines for recipients of NIH research grants and contracts on obtaining and disseminating biomedical research resources: final notice. *Fed Reg.* 1999;64(246): 72090-72096. http://www.ott.nih.gov/pdfs/64FR72090.pdf. Accessed April 15, 2013.
39. Office of Extramural Research. NIH Sharing Policies and Related Guidance on NIH-Funded Research Resources. National Institutes of Health. US Department of Health and Human Services. http://grants.nih.gov/grants/sharing.htm. Updated March 5, 2013. Accessed March 31, 2014.
40. Simon BM. How to get a fair share: IP policies for publicly supported biobanks. *Stanf J Law Sci Policy.* 2009;1:65-79.
41. National Institutes of Health. Final NIH Statement on Sharing Research Data. http://grants.nih.gov/grants/guide/notice-files/NOT-OD-03-032.html. Published February 26, 2003. Accessed March 31, 2014.
42. Office of Extramural Research. NIH Data Sharing Policy. National Institutes of Health. US Department of Health and Human Services. http://grants.nih.gov/grants/policy/data_sharing/. Updated April 17, 2007. Accessed March 31, 2014.
43. Bayh-Dole Act. PL 96-517, codified as 35 USC §§200-212, implemented by 37 CFR. 401. http://www.gpo.gov/fdsys/pkg/USCODE-2011-title35/pdf/USCODE-2011-title35-partII-chap18.pdf. Accessed April 15, 2013.
44. The Bayh-Dole Act: A Guide to the Law and Implementing Regulations. Council on Government Relations. October 1999. www.cptech.org/ip/health/bd/Bayh_Dole.pdf. Accessed April 11, 2012.
45. Ginsburg GS, Burke TW, Febbo P. Centralized biorepositories for genetic and genomic research. *JAMA.* 2008;299(11):1359-1361.
46. Clark BJ. Why goodwill alone won't work in biobanking initiatives. *ACP News.* Winter 2007:28-29. http://www.oncoreuk.org/pages/documents/ACPwinter-07articleonly.pdf. Accessed December 12, 2011.
47. Hunter P. More is less. *EMBO Reports.* 2007;8(7):626-628.
48. Bouchard RA, Lemmens T. Privatizing biomedical research: a "third way." *Nat Biotechnol.* 2008;26(1):31-36.
49. Recommendations of the caHUB Partnerships Group: making phase II possible. Report in preparation.
50. Vaught J, Rogers J, Myers K, et al. An NCI perspective on creating sustainable biospecimen resources. *J Natl Cancer Inst Monogr.* 2011(42):1-7
51. Vaught J, Kelly A, Hewitt R. A review of international biobanks and networks: success factors and key benchmarks. *Biopreserv Biobank.* 2009;7(3):143-150.
52. Huff C. Precious tumor: what happens to cancer tissue and why it's so valuable to researchers. *Cure.* June 10, 2007. http://www.curetoday.com/index.cfm/fuseaction/article.showArticleByTumorType/id/821/tumorCategory/Myeloma/article_id/190. Accessed March 31, 2014.
53. Waltz E. Tracking down tissues. *Nat Biotechnol.* 2007;25(11):1204-1206.

Disclaimer

The opinions expressed in this chapter are the authors' own and do not represent the official views of the National Human Genome Research Institute, the National Institutes of Health, the Department of Health and Human Services, or Deloitte Consulting.

Index

Web Resources

American Association for Cancer Research (AACR): www.aacr.org

American Society for Clinical Pathology (ASCP): ascp.org

American Society of Clinical Oncology (ASCO): www.asco.org

BBRB Biospecimen Research Database (BRD): brd.nci.nih.gov/

Biobanking and Biomolecular Resources Research Infrastructure (BBMRI): bbmri.eu

BioCoR Resources: biocor.umn.edu/biocor-resources

BioPortal: bioportal.bioontology.org

Biorepositories and Biospecimen Research Branch (BBRB): biospecimens.cancer.gov

Biospecimen Research Network (BRN): http://biospecimens.cancer.gov/researchnetwork/

Center for Biomedical Informatics and Information Technology (CBIIT): cbiit.nci.nih.gov

Centers for Medicare and Medicaid Services (CMS): www.cms.gov

Clinical Trials and Human Subject Protection, Food and Drug Administration: http://www.fda.gov/ScienceResearch/SpecialTopics/RunningClinicalTrials/default.htm

Collaborative Institutional Training Initiative (CITI): https://www.citiprogram.org/Default.asp

College of American Pathologists (CAP): cap.org

Cooperative Human Tissue Network (CHTN): www.chtn.nci.nih.gov

Enterprise Vocabulary Services (EVS): evs.nci.nih.gov

European, Middle Eastern and African Society for Biopreservation and Biobanking (ESBB): www.esbb.org

Good Laboratory and Manufacturing Practices: http://www.qualityassociatesinc.com/

Health Insurance Portability and Accountability Act (HIPAA): www.hhs.gov/ocr/privacy

Human Genome Organisation (HUGO): hugo-international.org

International Air Transport Association (IATA): http://www.iata.org/training

International Civil Aviation Organization (ICAO): http://www.icao.int/Pages/default.aspx

International Society for Biological and Environmental Repositories (ISBER): www.isber.org

National Cancer Institute (NCI): www.cancer.gov

Office for Human Research Protections (OHRP): http://www.hhs.gov/ohrp

OHRP Guidance on Research Involving Coded Private Information or Biological Specimens: http://www.hhs.gov/ohrp/policy/cdebiol.html

Protecting Human Research Participants, NIH Office of Extramural Research: http://phrp.nihtraining.com/users/login.php

Translational Research Program (TRP), SPORE grants: trp.cancer.gov

United States and Canadian Academy of Pathology (USCAP): www.uscap.org

United States Department of Transportation: www.dot.gov

US Department of Health and Human Services (HHS): www.hhs.gov

US Food and Drug Administration (FDA): www.fda.gov

World Health Organization (WHO): www.who.int

cap
PRESS

Also From CAP Press

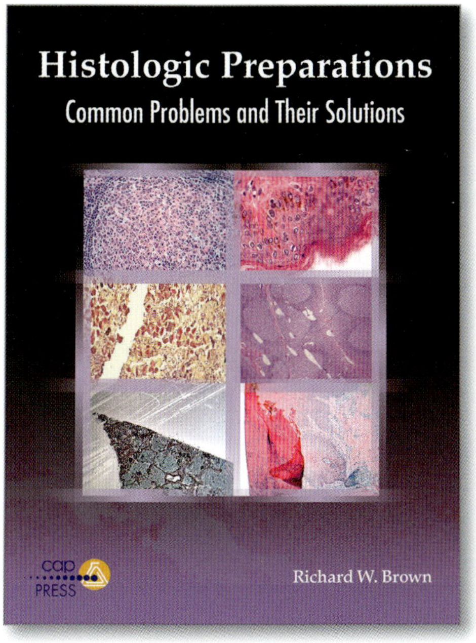

Histologic Preparations: Common Problems and Their Solutions contains troubleshooting techniques for the most common artifacts and problems incurred in routine histologic preparations. Developed by the CAP Histotechnology Committee in conjunction with the National Society for Histotechnology, it serves as both a reference text and teaching tool. Contents include:

- Fixation and processing
- Microtomy
- Frozen sections
- Hematoxylin and eosin
- Gram stain
- Mycobacteria, *H pylori,* spirochetes, and fungi
- Trichrome stains
- Reticulin
- Elastin stains
- Basement membrane
- Mucin stains
- Amyloid
- Immunohistochemistry

Softcover; 168 pages; 2009
Item: PUB123
List Price: $50
CAP Member Price: $40
Ebook Price: $37

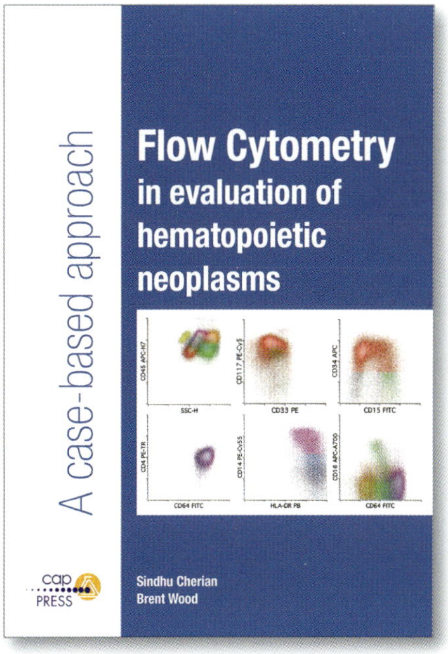

Flow Cytometry in Evaluation of Hematopoietic Neoplasms: A Case-Based Approach is a practical guide to flow cytometric analysis in the workup of hematopoietic neoplasms presenting in the peripheral blood, marrow, lymphoid tissue, and extranodal sites. Using multicolor techniques pioneered by Brent Wood, the text demonstrates a unique approach to diagnosis of malignancies as well as identification of small abnormal populations in the posttherapy setting (minimal residual disease testing). Contents include:

- Immunophenotypic changes seen in normal hematopoiesis
- Evaluation of lymphomas, leukemias, and myeloid stem-cell disorders
- A series of 36 cases, each dedicated to a specific disease entity, with detailed, full-color flow cytometric dot plots that clearly outline the features of the disease; a clinical history; and a thorough discussion, enabling readers to develop and work through a differential diagnosis and recognize diagnostic pitfalls
- Take-home points for each case

Hardcover; 176 pages; 2012
Item: PUB221
List Price: $110
CAP Member Price: $88
Ebook Price: $82

Also From CAP Press

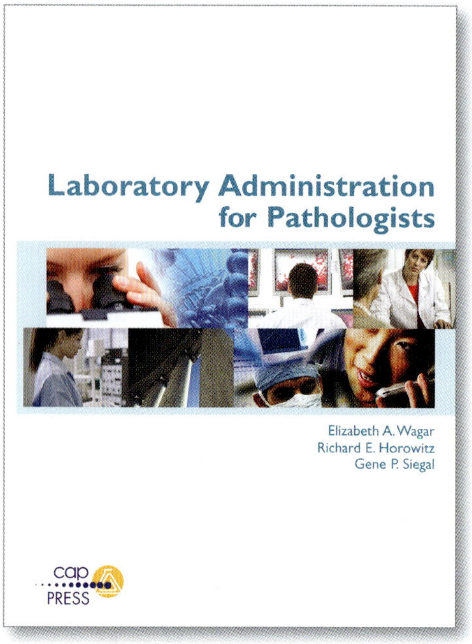

Laboratory Administration for Pathologists provides the core principles and tools of management for the practice of pathology and laboratory medicine. The book covers all aspects of clinical and anatomic pathology laboratory administration and is especially geared for trainees and young pathologists entering the field. Pathologists will find this text to be useful as a quick reference tool or to review management for maintenance of certification. Residents will find this text useful for board preparation and in rotations related to management training. Contents include:

- Management principles
- Competencies and interfaces of the involved pathologist
- Laboratory operations and personnel management
- Equipment and supplies, space planning, and laboratory information systems
- Quality management in laboratory medicine and anatomic pathology
- Financial management of the laboratory
- Laboratory laws and regulations
- Ethics for pathology and laboratory medicine

Hardcover; 300 pages; 2011
Item: PUB312
List Price: $100
CAP Member Price: $80
Ebook Price: $75

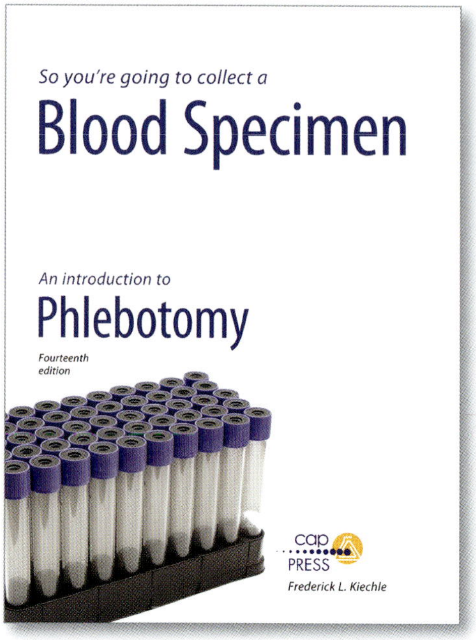

So You're Going to Collect a Blood Specimen: An Introduction to Phlebotomy is a well-illustrated, functional reference guide with step-by-step instructions for obtaining blood. Following these procedures will help minimize patient discomfort, ensure specimen integrity, and promote adequate protection against potential hazards of infectious disease. Contents include:

- Venipuncture from an arm vein
- Skin punctures in adults and children
- Blood smears and blood cultures
- Representative blood collection tubes
- Order of draw
- Specimen identification and labeling
- Standard precautions
- Sterility
- Disposal of used materials
- Quality assurance

Softcover, spiral bound; 80 pages; 2013
Item: PUB212
List Price: $25
CAP Member Price: $20
Ebook Price: $18
Volume discounts available on print version

To purchase a print book: cap.org, "Shop" tab
To purchase an ebook: ebooks.cap.org
Or call 1-800-323-4040 option 1

Prices subject to change.